Confessions of a Joyful Pharmacist

Tips, Tricks, Advice & Answers to Master Medications & the Pharmacy Experience

Ibiyemi Odetola Brown, Pharm.D.
Pharmacist, Wellness Coach, and Joy Scientist™

Six Joys Publishers

Atlanta

Confessions of a Joyful Pharmacist.

Six Joys Publishers.

The information contained in this book is for educational purposes only. It is based on research and the author's experience as a pharmacist; it is not a substitute for medical advice from your health care provider. The author and publisher do not endorse any products, medications, or services mentioned herein, and references made are simply used as examples only. All matters regarding your health require medical supervision. Consult your health care provider for health information specific to your care. Neither the author nor the publisher shall be liable or responsible for any alleged loss or damage from any individual, agency, business, or entity arising from information in this book.

Printed in the United States of America.

Library of Congress Control Number: 2021918436

ISBN: eBook: 978-1-7372441-2-7, print: 978-1-7372441-3-4

Dedication

To my mother, Ronke, the first pharmacist who sparked joy in me. Your ethical, professional standards and dedication as a health care provider inspired me to become a pharmacist, too. It is a true honor, sweet mother, to share a profession with a dynamic, amazing, and phenomenal woman like you.

To all my fellow pharmacists and all frontline community health care professionals, your value is immeasurable. Thank you.

To my parents, Dele and Ronke Odetola, who live a life of joy and gave me the gift of joy from birth that has resonated with me for my entire life.

To my brownies, Jake, Folasade, Olufela, Eniola, and Ayomide. And to my love, Eric Brown. You all sustain my joy every day.

To my grandmother, Francis Adebola Thomas, the thought of you fills me with transcendent joy.

And to Mimi—Cathey Brown. Your spirit lives forever in my heart.

With gratitude for the joys that surround me.

Acknowledgments

Thank you to all the pharmacists and pharmacy technicians who make many sacrifices for their patients every day. To all of the hardworking health care providers—nurses, doctors, technicians, and assistants-—thank you for your service and dedication to your patients. You are all Good Samaritans worthy of praise. You carry on despite the long hours, limited breaks, inadequate staff, and insufficient systems. The grit, passion, and resilience that you bring to your work every day is inspiring. Together, we must stay steadfast and not allow ourselves to get disillusioned. Together, we must continue to carry ourselves with dignity and professionalism. Together, we must remember that empathy is a key ingredient in patient care and endeavor to treat all patients with dignity and respect. Together, we must emerge from our comfort zones in patient rooms and behind the counter and share our stories. For too long, we have remained silent.

Contents

Preface

Do you take prescription medications or over the counter drugs? Do you care for someone who does? Do you visit the pharmacy or drug store once a while, occasionally, or very often?

If you've answered "Yes" to any of these questions, then this book is for you. As a patient who uses health care products and services, including drugs, you cannot afford to be passive about your health. You have to be proactive and stay informed. Gone are the days when patients could remain passive about their health problems. In the past, if you had a health problem or issue, you'd simply do the following: 1) go to the doctor, 2) get a prescription, 3) go to the pharmacist to get your medicine, 4) take your medication, and, finally, 5) get well. And that would be the end of it.

But in today's quickly-evolving health care climate, this process is unrealistic. Today, patients must become active participants in their health care decisions. If you don't, you are bound to have to deal with many frustrating encounters and end up wasting valuable time and money.

Although many health care decisions are made for us by health care providers and other third-party entities such as employers and insurance companies, there are still many choices we can make that directly affect our day-to-day lives. For example, you might get to choose your primary care doctor, health care specialists, insurance plan, and pharmacy. Knowledge is empowering, so be sure to inform yourself about those choices before you make them. They will have an impact on your health.

I have worked in the pharmaceutical health industry for nearly two decades. My journey from pharmacist to author was inspired by a desire to help patients better understand how to navigate through the confusion that often occurs when visiting the pharmacist. While it would seem that a trip to the pharmacy to pick up medication might be a quite simple and mundane undertaking, unanticipated issues can create a frustrating, even bizarre, experience. The pharmacist's conversation can be peppered with words like "formulary," "non-preferred," "deductible," "coverage gap," "prior authorization," and "generic substitution," sounding like a foreign language. The experience can be quite a challenge.

If that's true for you, you are not alone. I frequently encounter patients that haven't visited a pharmacy before or that are simply trying to pick up medications for a loved one or friend. I empathize with patients; I understand how perplexing conversations with a pharmacist can be sometimes. As the pharmacist, I often get the brunt of the frustration and blame for everything that could possibly go wrong. There I am, seemingly standing between the patient and their medications; it's not a position I want to be in. Yet, explaining to a patient why their insurance company denied their medication can be difficult and is often impossible.

Worse, if the pharmacist starts to use concepts that the patient has no knowledge of—at an emotional time, yet—it can make matters even more challenging.

I decided to write this book because I noticed that some patients leave the pharmacy with many questions still unanswered, and they might not fully understand the advice I gave them. I started to realize that many patients don't fully understand what pharmacists really do. They simply go to the pharmacist to pick up their medication; that is as deep as their knowledge goes. Since many people don't have the knowledge they need to make the process work for them, I want to provide that information.

In this book, I share over 17 years' worth of thoughts, experiences, and valuable health and wellness information that will enlighten you, save you money and time, and make your next trip to the pharmacy less stressful and intimidating. Think about it. If you had all the time in the world to ask your pharmacist all the questions you wanted to ask, what insights might you gain?

How to Make the Most of This Book

Confessions of a Joyful Pharmacist will help you begin to master an intricate mix of technical and practical concepts that will allow

you to navigate the pharmacy like a professional. To make the most of the book, pay close attention whenever you see the light bulb icon. This icon points out Quick Rx Tips that give you bite-sized bits of information that will be quick and easy to master. In addition, familiarize yourself with the Knowledge Checkpoints, which are located throughout the book to help you review, reflect, and clarify the material for yourself. The Knowledge Checkpoints give you a way to take notes for yourself and for discussions with your trusted pharmacist or health care provider, who can help you learn more about the nuances and standard protocols of their practice. This open dialogue with your pharmacist will be tremendously helpful as you navigate your medication and health needs.

Introduction

What does your health and well-being mean to you? What impact does it have on your life and relationships? How does it define you? Does it affect the way people see you?

These are questions that all of us might have to answer sooner or later. Your health affects your quality of life. While we all want to live long and healthy lives, illness can sometimes get in the way. Whether it is a sudden acute issue like a bacterial infection or a chronic health condition like heart disease, illness can disrupt your daily routine and rob you of quality time with your loved ones. It can affect you socially, physically, and mentally. It can also make you feel vulnerable and scared and leave you searching for solutions. Often, you will be dependent on others for assistance and for answers.

I know this from my own personal experience. I have lost beloved people in my life due to health issues. In 2016, my family lost our mother-in-law to pancreatic cancer, and even though time has passed, our feelings of loss are still very raw and difficult to accept. Then, in 2020, I lost my mother due to complications from acute gastritis. Sometimes it still feels like a dream; I keep thinking that, any day now, I will wake up and she will be with us again. But it never happens.

Our health and well-being can affect our relationships and, in turn, set the tone and the pace of our lives. As I reminisce about my childhood, I realize I never knew my paternal grandmother because she died when my father was a young child. I wish I had known her and often wonder what my life would have been like if she were alive. The same goes for my maternal grandfather, who died from cardiac arrest when I was a toddler. Although I did not get to experience life with them, I somehow know that my life would have been even richer with them in it.

As a pharmacist, I often speak to you from behind a counter, but I can relate to your health and life struggles. I, too, have had to navigate health emergencies for myself and my family. Whether it's taking a child to the emergency room after an accident, rushing to the pharmacy to pick up medications for a sick child, or taking care of a parent who had surgery, I have walked in your shoes. The everyday decisions we make impact our lives for the long haul, for better or worse, so informing ourselves about our health choices is extremely important.

Our health and well-being are deeply personal yet universal concerns. The potential for sickness is a concern of everyday life, whether it's a minor problem such as acid reflux, the common cold, or even a life-changing event like a cancer diagnosis. Often, medical science allows us to identify the cause of the sickness, treat the problem, and transition back to better and more wholesome health. For some, that transition can happen quickly, but for others, it can be a long and complex journey. Many times, illness is identified, but there is no known cure, and people have to cope with the trials of uncertainty. For many years, my husband has bravely navigated an incurable skin condition known as vitiligo. I find his resilience and the resilience of those who navigate life-altering diagnoses like his truly inspiring.

The Universal Need for Proper Care

The intended outcome of any health care system must be to provide the best possible health care solutions to meet the needs of its patients. Health care providers like myself have a responsibility to ensure that the treatments and services we provide to patients meet quality standards. As for medications, the World Health Organization (WHO), an international public health agency within the United Nations that advocates for patient health care needs around the world, recommends that patients receive "proper care," which they define as:[1]

- the right drug, which is the most appropriate for their condition
- the right dose, tailored to treat their symptoms
- the right duration that will resolve the health concern
- doing all of the above at the lowest possible cost to ensure affordability

Many countries, including the United States, continue to grapple with the intricate balance between these critical criteria. In America today, as more health care systems are run by private for-profit businesses, the challenge of keeping costs down continues to be a major issue. As we look to the future of health care in America, we should take stock of the wins while also addressing the systemic shortcomings of the health care sector. Is for-profit health care aligned to meet the needs of patients? Are not-for-profit systems capable of providing efficient health care on a large scale? What role should the government play in regulating the health care industry? According to The Centers for Medicare and Medicaid Services (CMS), health care spending is currently 17.9% of our gross domestic product (GDP), and, by 2026, it is projected to reach 19.7%.[2] The continued growth in health care spending is partly due to increased personal health-care spending, including higher premiums, higher deductibles, higher cost of brand name/specialty prescription drugs, and higher costs of medical care, products, and services.[3] The CMS also projects that by 2026, local, state and federal governments will finance 47%—nearly half—of all health care spending, up from the current rate of 45%.[4] Although many patients with insurance are still underinsured, one win we can celebrate is that access to health care has significantly improved, in part because of the passage of the Affordable Care Act. As of 2016, 91.1% of the American population was insured.[5] But even that number is projected to decrease to 89.3% by 2026.[6]

As a patient, the complexity of America's health care system requires you to ask questions, do your research, and be an active participant in your care. Doing so affords you a better health care experience. If you do not stay engaged, you might get the impression that the health care system is rigged against you. It is not a good feeling. But you can do something about it.

What Does a Pharmacist Do?

Today, the pharmacist is one of the most accessible health care providers you can find. You can literally walk into any community pharmacy around the country and speak to the pharmacist there without having to pay for a professional consultation. It is absolutely astonishing! Due to their knowledge, accessibility, and allegiance to the patient, pharmacists are continuously ranked among the top most-trusted professions.

A trained medications expert, a pharmacist has extensive knowledge of drugs and how they work in the body. While they do many things, their key role is to work with your doctor to make sure you get the best medication possible to help improve your health and quality of life. They check for contraindications, interactions, and compatibility, and they are also there to listen and answer your therapy questions and concerns. Just as importantly, they are there to offer positive reinforcement and to encourage you through your health care journey.

My job as a pharmacist does not end with helping patients with their medication needs, whether it be consoling a patient through loss, grief, or uncertainty, offering a shoulder to cry on, or lending an ear to simply listen. If a child got scratched up playing soccer, and Mom rushes over to the pharmacy for help, I clean the cut and bandage it up, putting a smile on the child's face. When a patient's medication was unavailable from the manufacturer, I took personal time to drive over to get their medication from another pharmacy, so they didn't have to go without needed medication. I've prevented a hypertensive crisis by performing a blood pressure check that saved a patient from a stroke. There are countless other stories like these that I can share, as do many other pharmacists.

A pharmacist serves in many capacities on the front lines of community care. We are counselors, nutritionists, insurance experts, medication experts, vaccine providers—and the list grows longer every day. We provide support to patients through sickness and health. We are visible in people's neighborhoods and hometowns across America. When patients have no medical home, when the doctor's office is closed, or when they cannot afford to seek care anywhere else, they come to us—their pharmacist. I wouldn't have it any other way. I love my job as a pharmacist, and it centers around joy. It is truly a joy for me to serve.

As a pharmacist, I like to connect deeply with my patients so that they feel like family. A few years ago, I lost a patient to cancer. It was an emotional journey caring for a patient with terminal cancer. I hoped and prayed for his recovery, and it seemed he was getting better. Unfortunately, he landed in hospice care after a stroke that he never fully recovered from. When I visited him, it broke my heart to see this once bubbly soul so frail. He could not speak anymore and communicated by scribbling short notes on paper. I sat by his side and talked to him, and he nodded and shook his head in response. Before I left, he scribbled a short note. "Thank you," he wrote. A few days later, I learned from his mother that he had passed away, and I wept. I attended his funeral and continue to remember him with the fondest of memories.

My journey as a pharmacist has taken me to many cities across Texas and Georgia. I have come across thousands of patients whose health care journey and pursuit of wellness inspires me every day. I am honored to have worked alongside talented teams of health care professionals whose mission is to help patients navigate their health journey.

We're in This Together

It is clear that the American health care industry has many flaws. If you have ever been a patient, as I have, you recognize that. We know that what often masks the systemic flaws is the hard work of the many health care professionals who care for patients. For our health care system to improve and rise to our expectations, we must speak up and share our experiences because patients will be the better for it.

If we are serious about making our health care system more efficient, we must all do the work. Patients must make informed choices and make it a priority to be active participants in their care. Our health care system today provides care that is not necessarily quality care. Common-sense reforms and solutions that should be bipartisan are politicized. We have lost the "sense" in common-sense reforms.

The unfortunate reality is that the cost of health care in America is beyond reach for many patients. People should not have to go bankrupt because of a medical condition or rely on charity to get simple dental procedures, medical care, or medicines. They should not have to resort to crowdfunding to finance health care costs or have to choose between paying rent and buying medications. Yet, that is often the case.

Until we get health care right as a nation, every health care provider will continue to bear the burden of caring for patients in a fractured and fragmented system. Every health care provider has to do the best they can with the resources they have. I've talked with providers for over 17 years, and many feel they do not have what they need to provide their patients with the best quality care. Health care providers can have the best intentions and be knowledgeable, highly skilled, and well-trained, but without adequate resources and effective systems, patient care suffers.

As a patient, it's important that you be vigilant and stay informed to create an optimal partnership with your health care provider.

It's a Joy

Being a pharmacist brings me a tremendous amount of joy. It is more than work for me; it is my true calling. I hope that the information you gain as you journey through these pages encourages you, educates you, and empowers you to become an informed consumer who is able to tackle your health decisions and engage in productive conversations with your pharmacist and health care providers. I hope to help you make your experience with your pharmacist a more informed, easy, and pleasant one!

The Oath of a Pharmacist

I vow to devote my professional life to the service of all humankind through the profession of pharmacy. I will consider the welfare of humanity and relief of human suffering my primary concerns. I will apply my knowledge, experience, and skills to the best of my ability to assure optimal drug therapy outcomes for the patients I serve. I will keep abreast of developments and maintain professional competency in my profession of pharmacy. I will maintain the highest principles of moral, ethical, and legal conduct. I will embrace and advocate change in the profession of pharmacy that improves patient care. I take these vows voluntarily with the full realization of the responsibility with which I am entrusted by the public.

Chapter 1
What You Don't Know About Pharmacists

Do you know what your pharmacist does every day? On a typical day in the pharmacy, your pharmacist is responsible for doing many things, including:

- providing health education and counseling patients about their prescriptions and over-the-counter medications.
- consulting with insurance companies to ensure correct billing, approval, and processing of prescriptions.
- providing a variety of health services, such as compounding, vaccinations, blood pressure monitoring, and health testing.
- dispensing medications, supplying drug labeling and medication guides, and transcribing doctor's orders into instructions that patients can readily understand.
- performing safety and quality checks to ensure the integrity of the medications.
- quarantining and returning medications that have been recalled by drug manufacturers.
- performing community outreach through wellness telephone checkups and health clinics.
- providing consultation services to health care providers involved in patient care.

- providing one-on-one medication management for patients with complex health and medication history.
- ordering medications from drug vendors, suppliers, and manufacturers.
- supervising and training other pharmacy care providers.
- transferring medications and medication records between pharmacies.
- performing drug finder services to help patients secure access to rare or specialty drugs.
- performing compliance audits for insurance and regulatory agencies.

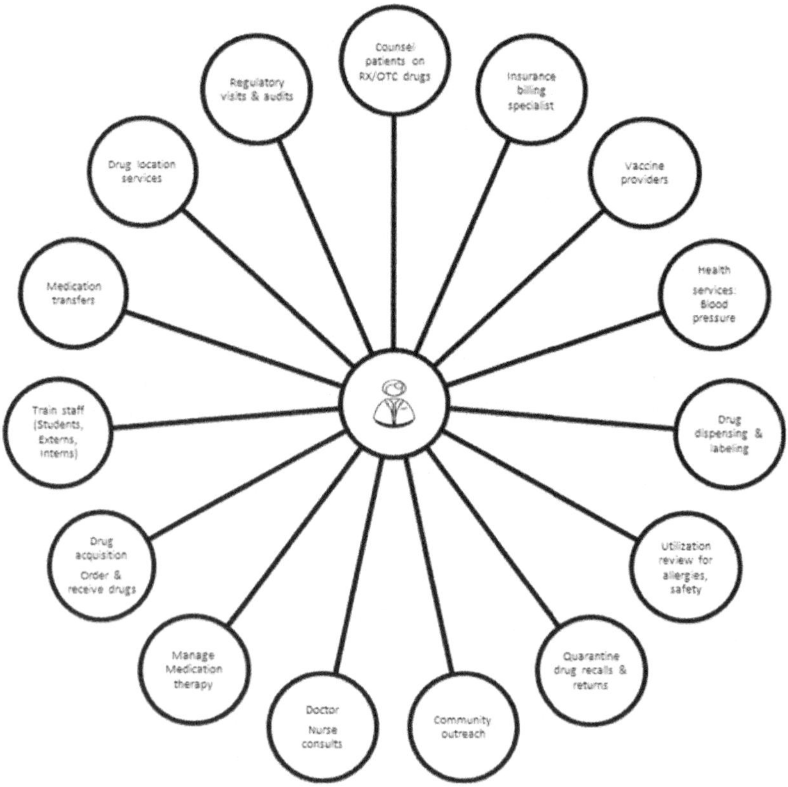

A Gallup poll ranks pharmacists among the top three most-trusted professions due to their honesty and ethical standards.[7] While you might not know it when you're in the pharmacy or talking over the phone, your pharmacist is hard at work performing essential safeguards on your behalf. They are contacting your doctor and insurance to get approval for your drugs; submitting prior authorizations to petition your insurance to cover your drugs; reviewing your chart for allergies, interactions, and dose appropriateness; and doing a whole lot more before your order ever gets filled. They do all that to ensure the safety of the medicines you consume.

We pharmacists take pride in doing everything that is humanly possible to help you get your medicine safely and understand how to take them. I love being a pharmacist. In our fragmented health care system, patients need an advocate looking out for them. We pharmacists do just that.

Helping patients make sense of their medication therapy is one of the sacred roles a pharmacist takes on. We are the true drug experts, the medication counselors, and educators. We wear our white coats with pride, and we've taken an oath to ensure the safety of our patients.

Community pharmacists are hardworking men and women who frequently face challenges such as being understaffed, under-equipped, overburdened, working long hours, and often having no scheduled breaks. I cannot begin to tell you how many times my lunch or dinner was left untouched because the pharmacy was so busy that I could not take a break, even to eat or to use the restroom. It is the love for my profession and patients that motivates and inspires me every day.

I hope that the valuable nugget of information you gain as you journey through these pages encourages you, educates you, and empowers you to become an informed consumer who is able to tackle your health decisions and engage in productive conversations with your pharmacist and health care providers.

For many aspects of our lives, technology affords us the luxury of getting things done quickly, and in the health care industry, technology often helps make health services delivery faster and more efficient. In fact, technology is integrated into most aspects of health care—medicine, surgery, ultrasound, medical devices, and laboratory testing. Though computers and technology in health care afford us the ability to perform complex and sophisticated tasks, ultimately, the human behind the machine is what brings it all together. As consumers, though, sometimes we conveniently forget that it is the trained medical professional—the human—who will interpret, analyze, and use the information to better care for us. Acknowledging this fact is important as we navigate the health system.

Take the pharmacist, for example. When a pharmacist receives a prescription order from a doctor, they will interpret, analyze, and use the patient's specific parameters—such as weight, allergies, health condition, and current drug regimen—to ensure that the prescription is safe before it is dispensed to you. Often oblivious to this chain of events, patients often assume that because technology is involved, these critical checks and balances that the pharmacist performs can be bypassed. But that is not the case.

Part of being an informed consumer is being able to tell fact from fiction. Yet, in an age when misinformation and false advertising are used for profit, it can sometimes be hard to do. For example, years ago, I heard an ad on the radio for a pharmacy guaranteeing that they would have prescriptions ready for patients in under 15 minutes. The ad went on to say that if the pharmacy took more than 15 minutes to fill a prescription, the patient would receive a gift card as compensation. But the reality for a pharmacist is that medications often take longer than 15 minutes to prepare.

I wish that patients wouldn't fall for those kind of cheap marketing stunts, but the unfortunate reality is that they do. Catchy ads with misinformation, though frivolous, have a way of etching themselves into our psyches. They often oversimplify the crucial roles of health care professionals. In our minds, we rationalize it; unconsciously, it becomes real and acceptable. The damage is done. The now-not-later attitude is an awkward but true reality in my profession. Often patients want us to complete their prescription order within seconds—as if they were in a fast-food drive-through lane. This creates a dilemma for the pharmacist because it is close to impossible to deliver quality care to patients using a model similar to that of a fast-food restaurant.

The Reality of the Wait

The unfortunate reality of a community pharmacy is that you simply need to be prepared to wait your turn to receive the services you need. You can wait for prescriptions you've dropped off, wait to pick up your prescription, wait to get your flu shot, wait to speak with the pharmacist, wait for your insurance to approve your medicine, wait for the doctor to approve your medication refill, and wait on the phone to get personal assistance. While all of that waiting is frustrating for patients, it is also frustrating for pharmacists. We don't want sick patients to have to deal with extended wait times just to get their needed drugs, either. But unfortunately, that is how our community pharmacy health system currently functions.

Why all the waiting? The wait is necessary because the same person that is checking you out at the register is the one that is filling your medicines, calling your insurance, ordering your medicines, answering the phones, working the drive-through window, and helping Grandma Jo find her vitamins. The next time you go to the pharmacy, pay close attention to the number of staff working behind the counter. Then ask yourself if that number is practical. Many community pharmacies across the country are seriously understaffed and ill-equipped to meet the expected needs of the patients they serve. With the accelerated expansion of large, corporate-run pharmacies, operational decisions that should be made by pharmacists—since they are much more in tune with their patients' needs—are being made by executives far removed from the pharmacist-patient dynamic. As a result, pharmacies in our communities are overwhelmed and unable to provide the high-level quality care that is expected of a 21st-century health care system. So, like so many other pharmacists, pharmacy technicians, and health care specialists across the country, they do the best they can with the resources at hand.

Of course, prescription medicine orders calling for an immediate turnaround have their place. Pain medicine following surgery, hypertensive medicine following release from the hospital, or antibiotics for an infection all needed to be filled ASAP. And your pharmacist will do everything feasible and safe to get your medicine order ready at a reasonable time. We are sincerely empathetic to patient's health and the need for urgency when it arises.

Quick Rx Tip: As a patient, you must understand that the pharmacist is required to review every single prescription for safety and accuracy before it is dispensed. There are NO exceptions.

Pharmacists perform essential safeguards that are critical to your care and safety; they cannot compromise that integrity. Pharmacists do not just "put a sticker on a bottle." On any given day, some patients might decide to stick around and wait for their prescriptions to be completed. Others choose to come back to pick up at a later time. Depending on the volume of prescriptions that have been submitted at the time you order yours, the wait times can vary. It might be quick and easy to process or take a little longer than expected. You will be given an estimate of how much time is needed to process and complete your medication order, as it often requires coordination and communication with your doctor and with your insurance carrier. Many other factors can affect the time it takes to complete your order, too.

For example, if you submitted your order of Lovastatin, your cholesterol medication, perhaps you were told it would be ready at 3 p.m. So you return at that time only to find out that your order is delayed. It's easy to be unhappy and get upset. But the wise thing to do is to have a productive conversation regarding the reason for the delay. You could also find out if you have other options if the wait appears to be too long.

A retail community pharmacy can sometimes be something like an emergency room: chaotic. At any given time, there are many moving parts. I sometimes find myself with doctor consults, patient consults, vaccinations to complete, drug vendors to check in, prescriptions to fill, patients to check in, patients to check out, a drive-through window to attend to, insurance consults, and a list of other issues to address—piling up, needing our attention.

One day, for example, I had five patients in the waiting area who were waiting for prescriptions that I was preparing for them; one of the patients was an infant that needed antibiotics for an infection. I had to call the insurance company to obtain pharmacy coverage information because the child's mother, who had active insurance, had not received her new card from her insurance plan. The little one's cries were deafening to everyone within earshot, and her mother was in a panic. So I took the time to calm her worries, and I stayed on the phone with the insurance company while they performed a coverage search. After a wait, they finally provided me with the coverage information needed to process the claim, allowing the mother to pay just a $5 copay instead of the $80 retail price for her child's medication.

This is what pharmacists do every single day for all of their patients, young and old. A community pharmacy typically does not have an onsite billing department that handles insurance claims; they usually have to resolve insurance benefit problems themselves. Other health care providers can retroactively bill for health services, or they have a designated onsite billing department. Retail pharmacy claims, however, are billed electronically soon after the prescription is received from the doctor or at the point a patient requests the prescription.

When you are waiting to pick up your medication, it's helpful to understand what has to be done before a medication can be dispensed and to remember that there might be other patients ahead of you that are sick and waiting too.

The Wrinkle with Insurance

People eventually discover that, regardless of the pharmacy they choose, there are many uncontrollable situations across the board that affect the supply and demand of medications. Insurance is one of them.

Your insurance policy determines if your insurance company will pay for your medicines and the terms of your coverage. Your pharmacy has no control over that.

A majority of Americans get their prescriptions from big box pharmacies that often have a one-size-fits-all model that is driven by sales and volume. Patients aren't privy to the extreme market forces that influence the pharmaceutical industry. Many factors, including consolidation, fluctuating pharmacy benefit reimbursement structures, moves to preferred provider networks, and ballooning drug prices, all contribute to slimmer profit margins for pharmacies nationwide. As a result, pharmacies end up doing more with fewer resources. In fact, the majority of pharmacies operate in the red, struggling day to day to break even. Many spend a lot to buy and store drug inventory in bulk, even though it might not get used. At the same time, pharmacies might not get fully reimbursed for the drugs that they do dispense to patients, and they end up with negative balance sheets.

Even with the challenges facing pharmacists, the best and most rewarding part of my job is the people I serve. Great experiences are routine for me! The joy I feel due to helping patients every day fuels my passion as a pharmacist and patient advocate. I have been hugged, kissed, and thanked. I have been praised and showered with love. I had one elderly patient surprisingly kiss me on the cheek because I took the time to make an over-the-counter drug recommendation. He had just had surgery to remove a small tumor on this face and was elated that the biopsy came back negative for cancer. Another patient returns to the pharmacy every month for his blood pressure medications and never fails to remind me that I saved his life. A few years earlier, he had come into the pharmacy, complaining of feeling "weird." I took his blood pressure, discovered it was dangerously high, and sent him to the emergency room. It was a close call.

My patients never hesitate to tell me how much they love and appreciate me. I have also had my share of grandma's chocolate cakes, cookies, and lemon pies. Many elderly patients come into the pharmacy by themselves. They tell me their kids and grandkids are not around; some of them don't have kids at all and live alone. I have become their confidante, health counselor, and drug counselor, and they come to me for many reasons, even some non-health-care-related concerns.

I make time for them. Many days, even in the midst of a chaotic day in the pharmacy, I'll step out to give them a hug, to talk to them, to counsel them, to console them, to listen to them, to pray with them, or to grief with them. In return, they thank me and tell me they love me. I live for those moments. As a health care provider, my patients are the greatest gift of joy.

Pharmacists do this kind of thing every day in communities and neighborhoods across America. Chances are, if your elderly loved one or parent lives alone or cares for themselves, they have a home away from home with their trusted neighborhood pharmacist, who takes care of their medication and health needs.

The Cost of Drugs These Days

As a patient, you should know the real costs of the drugs and health services you use. There is a huge difference between the actual costs of drugs and what you pay at the counter. When drug costs are subsidized or reimbursed by a third party, it is easy to get confused by the perceived costs. For example, a cholesterol medication you get every month at the pharmacy might only cost you a $5.00 copayment, but that is not the true cost. If you were to lose your insurance, you'd soon discover that the actual cost of the medication is $50. That's a big difference.

Another factor to keep in mind is that purchasing a more expensive brand name doesn't necessarily mean you'll get a better product; generics, although cheaper, are not necessarily less effective.

> **Quick Rx Tip:** With drug costs on the rise, if you want to cut costs on medication spending, you have to know your options and ask the right questions. Knowledge is power. The next time you take a trip to your pharmacy and are shocked by the high cost of your prescription, take a moment to process the information you are given and ask the right question, namely: What are my options?

It is easy to feel you have no control as a health care consumer, but you do have some control. The choices you make as a consumer have an impact on your health care costs, so it's best to be an informed consumer, take a proactive role in managing your health, optimizing your outcomes, and navigating the system. An uninformed patient will often end up been disappointed and paying more for care. You have to actively work to improve your health literacy; you cannot afford to be a naïve patient. Remember, the role of your health care provider is to assist you in your pursuit of a healthy living, but ultimately, you, the patient, are responsible for your day-to-day health and well-being. The time is now.

Begin today!

Chapter 2
Wellness 101: How to Spark Joy

Being a pharmacist brings me tremendous joy every day. That's true even if my work life can sometimes be chaotic and involve a hectic work schedule that requires multitasking, speed, and accuracy. I do all that while being on standby for patients, caregivers, prescribers, drug vendors, insurance reps, and many others! I realized at a young age that service to others is my passion, so I now choose every day to nurture joy in everything I do. I encourage you to do the same.

One day, I had a patient come in for an immunization consultation. I soon discovered that he was blind; he had lost his vision as an adult. So, after completing the vaccination, I helped him find some household items he needed. We talked for a few minutes, and I walked him to the exit to wait for his transportation. His kind and joyful demeanor had warmed my heart. He reminded me to seek joy in the simple things. He helped me realize that he could have approached his blindness with bitterness, but, instead, he chooses to live a life of joy in spite of his disability. As we said our goodbyes, he thanked me for my kindness.

My encounter with this man still resonates with me. Centering our lives around joy can be a prescription for true wellness. We can live a life of joy and meaning despite the odds!

One question that patients often ask me is what pill I recommend for mental health or happiness. “Help me find a pill that will make me feel good all day!” I often hear. When I dive deeper to get more insight about the person, I find that they are having a very difficult time coping with the many stressors they face in life. They are searching for tools and solutions to help them do a better job of balancing all aspects of their lives. I frequently get asked, both in my professional and my personal life, how I am able to stay calm and joyful even in the midst of disorder and chaos.

After all, just like you, I know stress. I stare chaos in the eye every day and have had my share of personal losses. But through it all, I choose to navigate the storm with mindful joy because it keeps me grounded and helps me cope with all of the stressors that come with life’s journey. But what I do have, I call the “joy perspective.” I inherited the joy perspective from my mother, who modeled a life of joy for me. Even in her last days, she stayed joyful. She was the very first pharmacist who sparked joy in me.

There is a science of well-being, and it offers invaluable insights into our quest for a healthier, more meaningful, and happier life. I use the science of well-being to stay grounded in my life, and it works. So, I call myself a “joy scientist” and choose to be it every day. I believe that you, too, have what it takes to become a joy scientist yourself.

What is a joy scientist? A joy scientist is simply someone who is passionate about sharing joy and uses the science of joy to enrich their lives and the lives of others. There are many simple ways to spark and sustain joy in your everyday life. The simple teachings of the practice can offer you the missing pieces that you can use, together with your medications, to be more healthy, both physically and mentally.

I know that a person's health care journey is usually not easy. There are many things to attend to, and taking medications is one of them. Yet while medications are often a very important part of one's healing process and recovery, the journey shouldn't end there. It is often the combination of medication and beneficial lifestyle practices that have the best healing effects on the body and mind.

Living a life of meaning and joy requires commitment and daily practice. It begins with very simple choices that you can incorporate into your life. You can begin to reap joyful rewards and experience joy today by using a few simple tools.

Simple Tools to Sparking Joy

1. Practice gratitude and show your appreciation for others, including strangers.

2. Practice kindness through your words and actions towards others, including strangers.

3. Get out in nature as often as you can. Being in nature and interacting with it is healing in itself.

4. Feed your body good nutrition. Make eating a variety of fruits and vegetables a priority.

5. Be conscious of your breathing. Practice deep, focused, abdominal breathing as often as you can.

6. Practice focused relaxation through simple muscle and body stretching exercises or activities.

7. Make it a habit to count your blessings every day by acknowledging and celebrating all of the joyful experiences and interactions you have.

8. Nurture your hobbies. Ask yourself: What activities do I enjoy? Then find ways to incorporate them into your routine. You may not have a lot of spare time, but a few minutes here and there are worth taking to savor your joys.

9. Volunteer your time, services, or resources to help others. For example, you might volunteer to read to children at a local library or make a dish for a potluck event at work.

10. Find ways to have a joyful perspective in your work life. After all, work life can sometimes be monotonous, chaotic, boring, challenging, fulfilling, and everything else in between! There are a lot of things about our work lives that we cannot change. So focus on what you can change in your work life, which is your perspective. Who says you can't take joy with you to work? Start by putting pictures of your loved ones at your desk or work station. Or perform simple acts of kindness by doing mundane things to help your clients or co-workers. A simple gesture from you can be extremely impactful for others.

11. Remember that sleep is *not* overrated. You need it. Make it a habit to get a good night's rest every day. Sleep is nature's "recharge and reset" button. In my opinion, a good night's sleep is better than any cup of coffee you ever had. And when you find yourself feeling tired, sleepy, or physically or mentally exhausted during the day, a simple, quick 15-minute power-nap can boost your energy reserves to get you through the rest of your day.

12. Practice meditation as often as you can. Meditation is a skill that you can develop and use over time. It does not have to be prolonged, nor do you need fancy equipment to be effective. Meditation is simply a mindfulness practice

that allows you to become more conscious of your thoughts. And since thoughts often affect our behaviors, meditation can be an invaluable tool to help us train our minds to focus and respond to positive and empowering thoughts. In turn, that can give us better control of our bodies and minds. There are many forms of meditation. Some use music, art, imagery, activities, and other objects. If you are new to meditation, keep it simple and find what works for you.

13. Prioritize people and experiences over material things. Material things may buy you comfort but will not sustain joy. As a young child, I grew up in Lagos, Nigeria, in West Africa. I did not grow up with the comforts of a microwave, washer and dryer, dishwasher, or access to 24/7 electricity or amenities. I took baths using a bucket of water. But guess what? When I look back on the 15 years that I lived there, I realize that they were filled with joy. The mere thought of my childhood lifts up my spirits with a transcending joy that is priceless.

14. Today is now! The past is gone, and the future will come. There is no moment like the present. Live in the present. It is easy to get caught up in the day-to-day hustle of life. Choose to stay present now! Staying mindfully present takes practice. Take it minute by minute, hour by hour, a moment at a time.

15. Learn to quiet the noisy distractions around you. From time to time, break away from the inevitable sensory overload and turn off your cellphone, television, gadgets, and electronics. Do a mental detox and unplug. Then, simply focus on you and your environment. Let yourself deeply experience the joy of simply being present where you are.

Where are you? Are you outside? What do you see? What do you hear? What do you feel? Marvel in the beauty that surrounds you. Notice the clouds, the sky, the birds, the trees, the flowers, the rain. Roll down your windows and take a breath of fresh air. Notice the person next to you. Whoever they are—family, friend, or stranger—engage them in conversation. Connect with them. Listen and build on actual social interactions.

16. Learn to have a generous spirit by performing random acts of kindness for people, including strangers. It can be as simple as holding the door or giving a compliment!

17. Find ways to share your joy. Make a list of the things that bring you joy and do them as often as possible. If you've included people on your list, write each of them a letter and tell them how much they bring joy to your life. Then, give them the letter in person or simply mail it to them. Watch your social bonds flourish.

18. Make a personal commitment to prioritize joy in your life. Joy is an integral part of wellness. When you practice joy often and make it a habit, it eventually becomes second nature to you. The more you nurture it, the healthier and more joyful you will be.

19. The science of joy is for everyone, young and old. It knows no limits or boundaries. And you can use it to cope with stress or whatever life throws your way.

20. Joy is the perfect gift; it is a gift that keeps on giving. It is free to give and receive. It is easy to detect, easy to share, and easy to spread. Together, as joy scientists, let's make joy go viral in our homes, workspaces, schools, businesses, and communities!

Chapter 3
So, You're Sick!

When you get sick, sometimes you wonder if your illness is bad enough that you should see a doctor or if you can safely self-manage. In the case of a life-threatening emergency, you should definitely seek emergency attention immediately. Self-management, on the other hand, is appropriate for minor issues such as the common cold, allergies, and minor aches and pains. There are many self-care, over-the-counter drugs and products that are available at the pharmacy for which you don't need a prescription from your doctor.

Self-management refers to a self-care regimen you might use to treat ailments and conditions on your own or with guidance from your health care provider. Self-care products are part of a multibillion-dollar industry that will continue to grow as patients become more active participants in their health care. Self-care can be safe and effective as long as people make educated and informed selections and follow the recommended package instructions. But self-management does not only have to do with medications; it can also include lifestyle changes and self-awareness strategies that are an important part of becoming a healthier person. Healthy nutrition, for example, plays an important role in the management of your illness and should be a part of your therapeutic plan. Taking ownership of your health by incorporating self-management routines, no matter how simple, can complement your existing medication regimen and can have positive results on your health.

Our psyches have a huge effect on our well-being, and how we perceive our health can affect our health outcomes. Patients who take control of their health and are actively involved in their health care will likely fare much better than those with a sedentary or passive approach. But always ask for answers from your health care providers whenever you are not confident and clear about your treatment plan or what you should be doing.

Here are a few conditions along with simple steps you can take to manage them:

Diabetes

Diabetes is a disease that results in high levels of sugar in the blood. Those who live with diabetes are encouraged to monitor their blood sugar levels to make sure it is at healthy levels. Supplies that allow you to check your blood sugar are available at the pharmacy and do not require a doctor's prescription. If you have health insurance, your diabetic testing supplies, such as blood glucose meters, test strips, and lancets, might be covered by your insurance plan with a doctor's prescription.

Gout

Gout is a disease that results in high levels of uric acid in the blood, which can crystalize and cause excruciating pain in and around joints throughout the body. Those who live with gout are encouraged to make dietary changes, eliminating foods that can increase uric acid levels, such as red meat and alcohol.

Chronic Pain

Pain is a very subjective experience. Chronic pain can result from a chronic disease, or it can be the result of pain that lingers long after recovery from an acute injury.

Patients living with chronic pain might benefit from incorporating complementary therapies such as physical and massage therapy, acupuncture, meditation, yoga, or Tai Chi into their medication treatment plan. Today, about four out of ten adults make use of complementary therapies.[8] They are most frequently used for back pain, neck pain, joint pain, muscle pain, arthritis, anxiety, cholesterol, common cold, migraines, and insomnia.[9]

Hypertension

Hypertension, also known as high blood pressure, is a disease characterized by an abnormal increase in the pressure of blood as it flows through blood vessels into and out of the heart. Those who live with high blood pressure are encouraged to monitor their blood pressure using a personal home blood pressure machine that is available at the pharmacy without a prescription from the doctor. Monitoring your blood pressure at home enables you to better manage and coordinate your care with your doctor.

Reducing consumption of dietary salt is often recommended for managing high blood pressure.

The Common Cold

The common cold is a syndrome caused by a viral infection of the nose and throat. Symptoms can include sore throat, cough, sneezing, runny nose, chest and nasal congestion, aches, and pains. Over-the-counter medications can help ease symptoms, but there is no cure for the common cold. Most patients self-manage using over-the-counter medications and complementary remedies.

Rubbing a vaporizing menthol and eucalyptus ointment on the body can be soothing for the common cold.

A warm cup of water with a hint of honey and lemon can soothe an aching throat.

Getting plenty of rest and hydration supports your immune system in the healing process.

If you decide to self-manage when you are sick, and your symptoms do not improve or become worse, consulting with a doctor is the right thing to do.

So, You Want To See a Doctor. Now What?

Patients often ask me how they might find a qualified health care provider. Here are several suggestions:

You can ask for referrals from friends or family. My children's pediatrician was referred to me by a colleague 14 years ago, and my kids still use the same doctor now. Everyone needs a primary care physician to monitor their health and wellness.

If you already have a primary care physician or other health care provider, you can simply ask for a referral, especially if you are seeking the services of a specialist. Doctors often work within networks of larger health care groups, so they can easily refer you to a provider for specialized care.

You can also use your insurance company's online database as a resource. There, you can use specific search criteria to find a provider that fits your needs. Some insurance companies also offer a health care companion service, providing you with personalized help to locate a doctor or specific service that meets your needs.

Community clinics in your county can also be a helpful resource. Hospitals and non-profit health organizations often provide outpatient clinical services in the local community they serve.

When you begin working with a health care provider, the goal is twofold: to diagnose—i.e., to get to the root cause of the problem—and to treat, meaning, to tailor a treatment plan to resolve or manage the problem. Access to quality health care resources is very important, but for many patients, it can still be a challenge. If you have health insurance, access to a health care provider is as simple as calling and scheduling an appointment or simply walking in. If you are without insurance, there might be more barriers in the way of getting help. Due to limited financial resources, many patients without insurance use the emergency room or urgent care facility. Health care costs are significantly higher than the average person can afford in general, and, for the uninsured, they are even more costly.

The Burden of Payment

Patients' wallets are taking a big hit these days. The cost of health care has become a burden for many homes; a whopping 62% of Americans seek bankruptcy protection because of health care costs.[10] With a household of four young children, I can relate to the constant cycle of unavoidable doctor visits and the challenges of paying off major medical bills in spite of having insurance. Even though I'm a pharmacist with health insurance, health care is still costly. At the same time, health care is becoming less sustainable for stakeholders such as insurance companies, employers, and health systems, and more of the cost burden is getting shifted to patients.

To be sick and unable to shoulder the cost of the services required to get you better can be an extremely overwhelming and dehumanizing experience. I've been through it. Years ago, when my family moved to Georgia, I started a new job, and there was a waiting period before my new health insurance benefits would kick in. But my infant daughter was sick and needed to see a doctor. When we got to the doctor's office, I was told to pay an outrageous amount upfront, an amount I didn't have, before the doctor could see my daughter. I pleaded with them to accept a partial payment up front and be billed for the remainder, but I was refused. I asked to speak to the office manager, and we agreed that I would pay half of the amount upfront and then be billed for the balance. While it makes perfect sense that providers should be paid their money upfront, the arrangement often puts patients between a rock and a hard place. Making matters worse, health care institutions often send unpaid medical bills to collections and even sue patients in court. It's like adding salt to an open wound.

Many private providers can require full payment for services rendered at a visit. If you are insured, it means that you have to pay a copayment or coinsurance. If you are not insured, the amount might be a lot more than you can afford. If you do not have insurance, ask about setting up a payment plan that allows you to pay in installments or about available discounts for uninsured patients. You can also look for community clinics in your area that provide health care services at lower costs.

When you visit a doctor for the first time, you will need to provide a complete medical, allergy, and drug history. Be as thorough as possible so that they get a full picture of your health status and so can better diagnose and treat the problem. Bring your Medication List, too. The doctor will ask you questions and might perform important examinations and assessments. They might want you to get additional labs or other tests to help with diagnosis and treatment. Before the end of your doctor's visit, make sure that you have a clear understanding of your treatment plan and what your next steps are. Do not be afraid to ask questions.

Since that white coat can be intimidating to some patients, write down your questions before your visit. (This is a perfect time to review and bring with you the notes you wrote down in the Consult sections of the Knowledge Checkpoints throughout this book!) Take a pen and notebook with you so you can write down important notes when you're there. If the doctor makes any changes to your medications, be sure you understand exactly what those changes are. Be certain about which medicines you are starting, discontinuing, or adjusting.

Making the Most of Your Doctor Visit

The doctor might prescribe a medicine for you and write you a paper prescription. The written prescription is a legal document that is issued and signed by the prescribing doctor to authorize a pharmacist to dispense medication to the patient. This prescription contains important information about your medication order. You then take your prescription to the pharmacy, where the pharmacist reviews it, prepares it, and dispenses your medicine to you.

Sometimes patients get confused when their doctor makes changes to their medicines. Then they come to the pharmacy, expecting the pharmacist to answer questions such as: "Does my doctor want me to continue or stop this medicine?" Unless your doctor makes such changes in writing and documents them on your prescription order, the pharmacist won't know about them. So while you are in your doctor's office, be sure that your doctor is putting their changes in writing.

If you have a chronic health condition such as high blood pressure, high cholesterol, asthma, or diabetes, your doctor will monitor your health condition and will likely require that you make routine, scheduled follow-up appointments. It is important that you keep all your doctor appointments to ensure the continuity of your care and your prescriptions. Your doctor might deny your prescription refill request in the future if you fail to keep up with your routine visits. If you miss an appointment with your doctor, be sure to reschedule as soon as possible to prevent disruption of your therapy.

Acute conditions such as minor bacterial or viral infections might not require a follow-up visit. Your doctor will inform you when they want to see you back in the office. Sometimes, the doctor might refer you to a specialist for further evaluation. And if you get discharged from a hospital or inpatient facility, you might be instructed to follow up with your primary care physician (PCP) or a specialist. Prior to discharge, make sure that you fully understand your take-home instructions, and then, of course, be sure to follow through with them!

Your pharmacist does provide an important check-and-balance service within the health care system. We are medical professionals who have been trained to know about drugs and drug therapy, and we are able to guide your doctor in selecting the right drug for you. Your pharmacist will review your medicine for safety and dispense it to you with instructions.

Your pharmacy will give you a customized drug information package that includes details about your medication and how to use it. Also, while you are in the pharmacy, you will have the opportunity to talk with the pharmacist and ask questions about your medicine. It is important that you take the time to speak with them before, during, or after you check out, especially if you are starting a new medication.

In your journey through the health care system, you will come across many health care providers—doctors, nurses, dieticians, physical therapists, laboratory technicians, radiologists, and pharmacists. All of them have a role to play in your quest for diagnosis and treatment.

Clarity Is Key

Ask questions, speak up, and be heard. If you need someone to repeat the information, say so. Do not be intimidated or afraid to speak up.

It's helpful to recognize that the American health care system can be disjointed and unorganized. It is unfortunately fragmented, and that fragmentation results in substantially higher costs. Every specialized medical professional involved in your care has to get reimbursed for their services. And the specialty health industry is booming because that is where the money is flowing. You might have an ear, nose, and throat doctor, an obstetrics doctor, a pain doctor, a gastroenterologist doctor, an eye doctor, a renal doctor, a dentist… and the list goes on.

In the real world, many patients find it hard to keep up with all of it. Since the system is disjointed, it can be easy for lapses in the continuity of care to occur. If you are seeing more than one doctor, you should make sure they *all* have updated medical records on file. Your doctors need to know what each other is prescribing so that dangerous duplications of medications and therapy does not occur. Good recordkeeping and organization on your part, as the patient, is key to making the system work best for you.

Quick Rx Tip: In all of your interactions, one key to getting good care is clarity. Be clear on the "what," "why," and "who" of your treatment or procedure. Use the 3W's technique to frame your health-related questions. Ask:

WHAT? *What* is this? *What* are you giving me? *What* am I receiving today?

WHY? *Why* are you giving me this? *Why* do I need this?

WHO? *Who* do I get this from? *Who* do I go to if I have questions? *Who* do I call for more information?

Knowledge Checkpoint

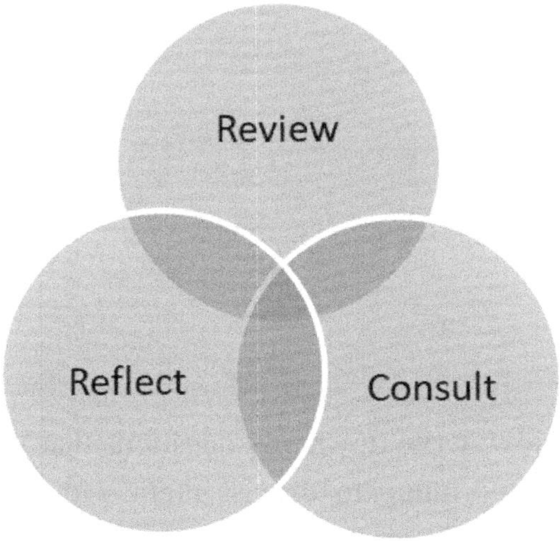

REVIEW: In the preceding three chapters, you learned more about pharmacists and the many ways they keep you safe and care for you. You have acquired an understanding of wellness tips that can help you develop a "joy perspective" and live a healthier, happier, and more balanced life. You have also learned about several self-management tips and best practices to guide you in accessing and navigating your care.

REFLECT: Take a moment to reflect on what you have learned and then answer these questions: How will you use the added insight to better navigate your health? What are you going to do from now on to incorporate more joy into your life? What steps are you going to take to better manage your present health care needs?

CONSULT: Now, write down any questions that you have. Then, take the next opportunity to discuss them with your health care provider and get the answers you need.

Chapter 4
Know Your Medications

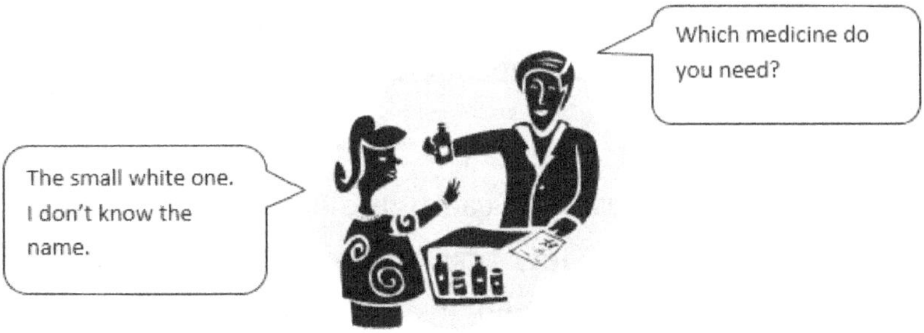

Many patients suffer from chronic health issues—such as heart disease, diabetes, depression, hypertension, osteoporosis, respiratory and thyroid disease—for which they take commonly prescribed medicines. But I cannot stress enough how important it is to know the names of the medications you're taking. Sure, many of them are hard to pronounce, and they can sometimes sound like gibberish. But the pharmacist will not mind if you mispronounce them. Butcher it if you want! But by all means, know what you are taking.

Drug Names

There is no doubt that pharmaceutical drug names can be confusing and can at times seem irrational. Trying to decipher drug names can leave patients stumped. Adding to the confusion is the fact that a single drug can be referred to by two different names: its generic name and its brand name. The *generic name* of a drug represents its molecular or active ingredient. A generic drug has the same active or pharmaceutical ingredient as the brand; it is approved for sale after the patent on the brand name drug expires. The *brand name* of a drug is the legal trade name of a drug for which a pharmaceutical company holds a patent, and it is decided by the drug company that manufactures it. Before a drug can be released to the public, it is required to have a generic name that helps categorize the therapeutic use of the drug.[11] The United States Adopted Names Council (USAN) assigns a generic name to drugs using embedded drug name stems that can help identify the drugs' classification and therapeutic use.[12]

Thankfully, there is a simple method for understanding complicated drug names. You can figure out what medications are and what they are used for, first by breaking down the generic name of the drug, and second, by recognizing simple prefixes, infixes, and suffixes that are embedded in the name. Drugs in a similar therapeutic class will often share common prefixes, infixes, or suffixes.

Some names have hidden clues to help you more easily identify and understand generic drug names. Here are a few to get acquainted with. Keep in mind that the following examples are simply guides; they are not absolute rules.

Drugs used to *lower cholesterol*, known as the "*statins*," might have "statin" at the end of the generic drug name. For example:

- Pravastatin
- Lovastatin
- Simvastatin
- Atorvastatin
- Rosuvastatin

Drugs used for pain and inflammation, such as non-steroidal anti-inflammatory drugs (*NSAIDS*), might have "*profen*" or "*proxen*" at the end of the name. For example:

- Ibuprofen
- Flurbiprofen
- Ketoprofen
- Naproxen

Drugs used to treat viral infections are known as *antiviral* drugs. They might have "*vir*" at the end of the generic name. For example:

- Acyclovir
- Valacyclovir
- Oseltamivir
- Norvir
- Famciclovir

Drugs used as *antibiotics* to treat bacterial infections might have "*mycin*" at the end of the name. For example:

- Azithromycin
- Clarithromycin
- Clindamycin
- Tobramycin
- Gentamicin
- Erythromycin
- Neomycin

Drugs used to treat *fungal infections* might have "*conazole*" or "*azole*" at the end of the generic drug name. For example:

- Clotrimazole
- Miconazole
- Fluconazole
- Itraconazole
- Ketoconazole
- Econazole

Drugs that are a *derivative of penicillin* are used to treat bacterial infections might have "*cillin*" at the end of the name. For example:

- Amoxicillin
- Amoxicillin/Clavulanate
- Ampicillin
- Dicloxacillin
- Penicillin

Drugs known as *quinolone antibiotics* are used to treat bacterial infections and might have a "*floxacin*" at the end of the generic drug name. For example:

- Ciprofloxacin
- Levofloxacin
- Ofloxacin
- Moxifloxacin
- Gatifloxacin

Drugs known as *tetracycline antibiotics* are used to treat bacterial infections and might have "*cycline*" at the end of the generic drug name. For example:

- Doxycycline
- Tetracycline
- Minocycline

Drugs that are a *derivative of codeine* and are used to treat pain might have "*codone*" or "*codeine*" in the generic drug name. For example:

- Hydrocodone
- Oxycodone
- Codeine
- Acetaminophen/Codeine
- Butalbital/Acetaminophen/Caffeine/Codeine

Drugs that are a *derivative of morphine* used to treat pain might have "*morph*" in the generic name. For example:

- Morphine
- Hydromorphone
- Oxymorphone

Drugs used as *beta-blockers* are used to treat high blood pressure and other health conditions. These drugs might have a "*lol*" at the end of the generic drug name. For example:

- Atenolol
- Bisoprolol
- Labetalol
- Nebivolol
- Sotalol
- Metoprolol
- Carvedilol

- Nadolol
- Propranolol

Drugs known as *angiotensin converting enzyme (ACE) inhibitors* are used to treat high blood pressure and other heart conditions and might have a "*pril*" at the end of the generic drug name. For example:

- Lisinopril
- Quinapril
- Captopril
- Enalapril
- Benazepril
- Fosinopril
- Ramipril

Drugs known as *angiotensin receptor blockers (ARBs)* are used to treat high blood pressure and other heart conditions. They might have "*sartan*" at the end of the generic drug name. For example:

- Valsartan
- Losartan
- Candesartan
- Olmesartan
- Telmisartan
- Irbesartan

Drugs known as *calcium channel blockers* are used to treat high blood pressure and other heart conditions. They might have "*dipine*" at the end of the generic name. For example:

- Amlodipine
- Nifedipine

- Nisoldipine
- Felodipine

Corticosteroids are a large family of drugs that are available in different formulations to treat many conditions. They might have "*asone*," "*cort*," or "*olone*" at the end of their name. For example:

- Hydrocortisone
- Betamethasone
- Dexamethasone
- Alclometasone
- Fluticasone
- Mometasone
- Fludrocortisone
- Triamcinolone
- Prednisolone
- Prednisone
- Methylprednisolone

Drugs known as *bisphosphonates* are used to prevent and treat osteoporosis (bone loss) and might have "*dronate*" at the end of the generic drug name. For example:

- Alendronate
- Risedronate
- Ibandronate

Drugs known as *proton pump inhibitors* are used to treat stomach acid reflux disease and might end in "*prazole*." For example:

- Omeprazole
- Lansoprazole

- Esomeprazole
- Rabeprazole
- Pantoprazole

Drugs known as *benzodiazepines* are used in the treatment of a range of neurological disorders. They might end with "*zolam*" or "*zepam*" in the generic drug name. For example:

- Alprazolam
- Clonazepam
- Triazolam
- Lorazepam
- Estazolam
- Diazepam
- Midazolam
- Flurazepam
- Temazepam
- Oxazepam

A group of drugs used to treat migraine headaches, known as the "*triptans*," will have "*triptan*" at the end of the generic drug name. For example:

- Sumatriptan
- Zolmitriptan
- Rizatriptan
- Eletriptan
- Frovatriptan
- Naratriptan

Drugs known as *antihistamines* can be used to treat allergies. These drugs might have derivatives of "*tadine*" in the generic name. For example:

- Loratadine
- Desloratadine
- Fexofenadine
- Olopatadine
- Cyproheptadine

Drugs used as *immune system suppressants* might have "*imus*" in the generic name. For example:

- Tacrolimus
- Sirolimus
- Pimecrolimus

Drugs derived from *sulfonamide*, also known as sulfa drugs, are used in the treatment of bacterial infections and might have "*sulfa*" in the generic name. For example:

- Sulfamethoxazole/Trimethoprim
- Sulfadiazine
- Sulfacetamide

Drugs used as *local anesthetics* for pain relief might have "*caine*" in the generic name. For example:

- Dibucaine
- Lidocaine
- Prilocaine

Drugs known as *fibrates* are used to lower triglyceride and cholesterol levels. They contain "*fibrate*" or "fibr" in the generic name. For example:

- Fenofibrate
- Gemfibrozil
- Fenofibric acid

Drugs used to treat *thyroid disease* might have "*thyro*" in the generic name. For example:

- Levothyroxine
- Liothyronine

Drugs used to *lower blood sugar* (glucose) levels might have "*formin,*" "*gli,*" "*glitazone,*" or "*gliptan*" in the generic name. For example:

- Metformin
- Glipizide
- Glimepiride
- Glyburide
- Pioglitazone
- Sitagliptan
- Linagliptin
- Saxagliptan

Drugs known as *cephalosporins* are a class of antibiotics used to treat bacterial infections. These drugs can have a derivative of "*cef*" in the generic name. For example:

- Cefdinir
- Cefepime

- Cephalexin
- Cefprozil
- Cefuroxime

Remember that drugs are classified under sub-categories based on how they work in the body. Your doctor uses specific patient criteria such as weight, age, allergies, symptom severity, and other factors such as kidney and liver function to determine which drug is safest to treat your condition.

> **Quick Rx Tip:** Always refer to your medication packet for detailed information on your medicine. The medication you receive might be a generic drug (nonproprietary) or a brand name (patented) drug. Listed in your medication packet is the generic or active ingredient name. At first glance, it might seem confusing or irrational, but if you look closer, you might find the clues that can help you better understand your medication classification and use.

The Most Common Prescription Drugs

The most commonly prescribed drugs constitute an interesting mix of medications and shed light on the most common health issues patients face today. Patients in the United States deal with a complex range of chronic health conditions, the leading ones being high blood pressure, diabetes, high cholesterol, pain, depression, anxiety, respiratory and, gastrointestinal diseases.

Some of the most commonly used prescription drugs in the U.S. include:

Acetaminophen/Codeine	treats pain
Albuterol	treats asthma symptoms
Alendronate	treats osteoporosis
Alprazolam	treats anxiety
Amlodipine	treats high blood pressure
Amoxicillin	treats bacterial infection
Amoxicillin/Clavulanate	treats bacterial infection
Aripiprazole	treats mood disorders
Aspirin	treats pain, fever and inflammation
Atenolol	treats high blood pressure
Atorvastatin	treats high cholesterol
Azithromycin	treats bacterial infection
Budesonide/Formoterol	treats asthma symptoms and chronic obstructive pulmonary disease
Bupropion	treats depression
Carisoprodol	muscle relaxant
Carvedilol	treats high blood pressure
Celecoxib	treats pain and arthritis
Cephalexin	treats bacterial infection
Cetirizine	treats allergies
Ciprofloxacin	treats bacterial infection
Citalopram	treats depression
Clonazepam	treats anxiety
Clonidine	treats high blood pressure
Clopidogrel	antiplatelet used to prevent blood clots

Cyclobenzaprine	muscle relaxant
Diclofenac	treats pain
Diltiazem	treats high blood pressure
Docusate	treats constipation
Donepezil	treats Alzheimer's
Duloxetine	treats depression
Enalapril	treats high blood pressure
Ergocalciferol	dietary vitamin D supplement
Escitalopram	treats depression
Esomeprazole	treats acid reflux
Ethinyl estradiol/Progesterone combinations	Contraceptive
Ezetimibe	treats high cholesterol
Ezetimibe/Simvastatin	treats high cholesterol
Fenofibrate	treats high cholesterol
Fexofenadine	treats allergies
Finasteride	treats benign prostate hyperplasia and hair loss
Fluconazole	treats fungal infection
Fluoxetine	treats depression
Fluticasone Propionate	treats seasonal allergies
Fluticasone/Salmeterol	treats asthma symptoms and chronic obstructive pulmonary disease
Furosemide	treats high blood pressure
Gabapentin	treats fibromyalgia
Glimepiride	treats diabetes
Glipizide	treats diabetes
Hydrochlorothiazide	treats high blood pressure

Hydrocodone/Acetaminophen	treats pain
Hydroxyzine	treats allergic reaction or itching
Ibuprofen	treats pain and inflammation
Insulin	treats diabetes
Lamotrigine	Anticonvulsant
Latanoprost	treats glaucoma
Levofloxacin	treats bacterial infection
Levothyroxine	treats thyroid disease
Lisinopril	treats high blood pressure
Lisinopril/Hydrochlorothiazide	treats high blood pressure
Loratadine	treats seasonal allergies
Lorazepam	treats anxiety
Losartan	treats high blood pressure
Lovastatin	treats high cholesterol
Meloxicam	treats pain and inflammation
Metformin	treats diabetes
Methylphenidate	treats attention deficit hyperactive disorder
Methylprednisolone	steroid used to treat conditions such as inflammation
Metoprolol Succinate	treats high blood pressure
Metoprolol tartrate	treats high blood pressure
Mometasone nasal	treats seasonal allergies
Montelukast	treats asthma and seasonal allergies
Naproxen	treats pain and inflammation
Omeprazole	treats acid reflux
Ondansetron	treats nausea
Oxycodone/Acetaminophen	treats pain
Pantoprazole	treats acid reflux

Pioglitazone	treats diabetes
Polymyxin	treats bacterial infection
Potassium Chloride	dietary potassium supplement
Pravastatin	treats high cholesterol
Prednisone	steroid treatment for inflammation and autoimmune conditions
Pregabalin	treats fibromyalgia
Promethazine	treats nausea
Propranolol	treats high blood pressure
Quetiapine	treats mood disorders
Rosuvastatin	treats high cholesterol
Sertraline	treats depression
Simvastatin	treats high cholesterol
Sitagliptin	treats diabetes
Spiriva	treats pulmonary disease
Spironolactone	treats high blood pressure
Sulfamethoxazole/Trimethoprim	treats bacterial infection
Tamsulosin	treats benign prostate hyperplasia
Topiramate	Anticonvulsant
Tramadol	treats pain
Trazodone	treats depression
Triamterene/Hydrochlorothiazide	treats high blood pressure
Valsartan	treats high blood pressure
Valsartan/Hydrochlorothiazide	treats high blood pressure
Venlafaxine	treats depression
Viagra	treats erectile dysfunction
Warfarin	anticoagulant used to prevent blood clots
Zolpidem	treats insomnia

Keep in mind that the treatments listed are not exhaustive and are provided only for educational purposes. Most prescription drugs have multiple uses.

Your Medication List

Be sure to keep a written record of your current medications, both your prescription medications and what you buy over the counter in your own personal list of medications. Document the dose you take, the reason you're taking it, and the prescribing doctor. Then, update your Medication List any time your doctor changes your dosage, stops a medication, or starts you on a new one. Be sure to put your Medication List somewhere that is easy to access, such as in a wallet or on a mobile phone. It will be immensely valuable to help you stay organized and track which medications you need whenever you request a refill from your doctor or pharmacist.

Quick Rx Tip: A pharmacy can house hundreds and thousands of prescription and over-the-counter medications. Referring to your medication in vague terms like "the small blue tablet" or "the round red pill" is not safe and can lead to serious medication errors. When in doubt, use your prescription bottle, refill number, or medication list to reference or request the specific medication you need.

Your Medication List will contain valuable information that you might need to provide to your health care provider, especially if you have more than one doctor you're working with. You might also need it if you go to the hospital or an inpatient facility. When it is complete and up to date, your list helps you ensure there's a smooth continuity of care. It can also prevent medication errors.

Your Medication List should contain the names of the medications you take, how you take them, what you take them for, and the name and contact information of the prescribing doctor. It is also a good idea to include the date that your list was prepared or updated. Here's an example:

Jane Doe

My Medication List **Current as of May 25, 2021**

Medication	Dose	Indication	Doctor/Phone
Metoprolol tartrate 25mg	1 tablet twice a day	Blood pressure	Dr. Elly 555-555-5555
Simvastatin 40mg	1 tablet daily at bedtime	Cholesterol	Dr. Elly 555-555-5555
Latanoprost 0.005% Eye drops	1 drop in both eyes at bedtime	Glaucoma	Dr. Foxy 222-222-2222
Aspirin 81mg	1 tablet daily	Anticoagulant	Dr. Elly 555-555-5555
Metformin 500mg	1 tablet twice a day with meals	Diabetes	Dr. Johnson 777-777-7777
Tylenol 500mg	1 tablet every 4 to 6 hours when needed	Pain	Over the counter

Chapter 5
A Day in the Life of a Pharmacist

We pharmacists are some of the most valuable and accessible of all health care providers available to you. We are medication experts that provide you and your doctor with information that helps you make informed decisions about your medicines. We help you make sense of your medications, ensure that you get the right medication and the right dose, and screen for potential interactions with your other medications.

Your pharmacist has gone through intensive training and is highly knowledgeable in the science of medicine. Pharmacists today graduate with a clinically focused Doctor of Pharmacy degree (Pharm. D.) and are the most qualified health care providers when it comes to drug information. Your pharmacist doesn't just fill your prescriptions; they perform certain clinical functions, depending on their setting. In the retail or outpatient setting, their services can include medication therapy management, blood pressure monitoring, diabetes and cholesterol screening, and immunizations. In a hospital or inpatient setting, pharmacists work on teams with doctors, dieticians, nurses, and other providers to improve patient therapy outcomes.

The role of a pharmacist has expanded, too; they are not merely a "pill counter" or dispenser of medications. They are often some combination of medication therapy experts, vaccine providers, drug and health information specialists, health education counselors, patient and public health advocates, COVID-19 specialists, and much more!

But one thing that the pharmacist does not do is determine how much you pay for your prescriptions. Still, there are several things they *can* do to help you get the best price for your medicine. They can discuss the available medication alternatives that might be cheaper with you or your doctor. They can also direct you to drug coupons or prescription assistance programs that might be available to help lower the cost of your medication.

The pharmacist gets assistance from a *pharmacy technician* who performs data entry, prescription filling, and other technical and auxiliary functions.

A Typical Day in the Life of a Community Pharmacist

A pharmacist's day is usually jam-packed! A typical day usually includes:

- Reading notes from the previous day or the earlier shift, reviewing messages, reading emails, and mapping out priorities and follow-up duties for the day.
- Processing prescription orders and dispensing medications.
- Consulting with doctors to obtain refills, clarifying prescription orders, and requesting drug changes and prior authorizations.
- Checking in and putting up drug orders and shipments.
- Checking doctor's verbal, telephone, electronic, and faxed orders.
- Calling insurance companies to resolve any of the following: prescription issues relating to eligibility, early refills, quantity limits, cost limits, drug or formulation denials, and prior authorization requests.

- Providing vaccinations.
- Providing COVID-19 testing.
- Providing clinical services, including blood pressure, diabetes, and cholesterol screening.
- Quarantining expired and recalled drugs.
- Counseling patients and making medication recommendations.
- Checking in on patients through follow-up outreach calls.
- Performing drug search services by helping patients locate drugs that are needed immediately but not readily available.
- Transferring prescriptions to and from other pharmacies.
- Doing quality checks: reviewing each prescription for legitimacy, accuracy, and safety before it is sold.
- Ordering medications from pharmaceutical wholesalers for patients.
- Training pharmacy staff and overseeing students and interns educational learning.
- Resolving patients' medication issues and inquiries.
- Attending pharmacy operation meetings.
- As the need arises, assisting a patient that needs multiple medications today because they are traveling out of the country tomorrow. This involves calling their doctor and insurance company to get travel approval at the last minute for all their medications.
- Providing in-store help such as answering questions about where products are located in the aisles or doing price checks as requested.
- Checking out a patient's medicine, along with a cart-full of groceries, and sometimes waiting while they go search for a forgotten item.

- Listening to drug sales agents and drug discount card sales reps as they try to market their newest drugs.
- Dealing with occasional forged prescriptions. In a recent case, for example, the doctor's prescription pad had been stolen, and someone had been using it to forge prescriptions. The doctor wanted the person arrested.
- Showing a patient how to use the home blood-sugar monitor that they purchased.
- After closing the pharmacy, spending time cleaning, organizing, and working on projects.

Some True Stories

Events like these happen quite often—sometimes every day.

A patient came to the pharmacy requesting a refill on a medicine. The insurance denied the request because it was too early. The records showed that the patient had picked up his medicine a few days before, so he shouldn't have been out of them yet. I reprinted a copy of the receipt, which included a timestamp and payment details. The patient got angry and hysterical, insisting that he did not pick it up. I recommended that he go home and check again. A few hours later, he called the pharmacy and asked to talk to me. He had found his bottle of medicine and apologized for yelling at me. He had completely forgotten that he had picked it up already.

The printer stopped working, and I couldn't figure out what was wrong. I contacted the technical support team, and they told me that it would take a few hours to get it fixed. The backlog piled up, and many prescription orders were delayed. Patients (and pharmacists!) were impatient.

A patient walked in with his son and wanted me to look at the rash on his son's face and tell him what it is.

A patient came in and pointed out the high deductible that his insurance wanted him to pay for his medicine. He gave me several discount cards to try, but the price they quoted was more than the price of his medicine plus the deductible. His insurance company's offer was still the best price. He complained and called his insurance company. After an hour of trying everything, he realized there was nothing either one of us could do about his deductible. It took an hour at the consultation window for him to arrive at that conclusion.

A patient walked in needing a drug recommendation. She asked me to inspect the rash under her breasts, turned, and waved for me to follow her into the restroom to take a look.

A patient was unhappy because her medicine wasn't ready for her when she came to pick it up. We called the doctor's office to find out more and discovered that the doctor had called in the medicine to a different pharmacy. The patient had come to the wrong location.

A patient dropped off a prescription through the drive-through lane with a juicy burger in his hand. I hadn't eaten lunch yet, and the burger looked quite tasty. My stomach started to grumble from hunger pangs, and I felt the onset of a migraine coming on. I made a mental note to eat something soon. A few hours later, I stepped into the lunchroom to take a few minutes to eat something, but as soon as I started eating, I was paged to go back to the pharmacy. I scoffed down a few bites of food and headed back to work. On my way out the door at the end of the day, I remember I hadn't gotten to finish eating my lunch. My food was still sitting in the fridge in the lunchroom, barely touched.

❖

An elderly patient came in, distraught. She was visiting her family from out of town for a few weeks, but she had forgotten to bring all of her medicines. She was hard of hearing, too. She pleaded for my help. I reviewed the drugs she needed with her. She was well-organized and had with her a written list of all of her drugs, dosages, and even her doctor's phone number. She sat patiently in the waiting room as I went to work. I paged her doctor, who called back within minutes and gave me orders for her medicines. Then I spent another half hour on the phone with her insurance company to approve her travel supply. We were able to give her all the medicines she needed.

❖

A patient brought in his home blood pressure monitor. It wasn't working, and he wanted me to fix it.

❖

A patient brought in a couple of loose, unidentified pills that she found at home and wanted me to tell her what drugs they were.

❖

These are just a drop in the bucket of the never-boring events in a day of a hometown community pharmacist!

Chapter 6
Pharmacy 101

Drugstores and pharmacies are an essential component of the health care system. A pharmacy is where you go to get your medications or to get advice and information about medications. Drugstores are convenience stores that include a pharmacy, and they come in all shapes and sizes. Pharmacies can be local and independent, or they can be in grocery stores, supermarkets, mail-order businesses, clinics, and hospitals. They can be a compounding, specialty, or a corporate chain pharmacy.

Medicines obtained from a community pharmacy typically fall into three categories: prescription, over-the-counter, and behind-the-counter drugs.

Prescription (Rx) Drugs

Prescriptions can be written for medications, medical devices, or supplies that can only be dispensed and purchased with a valid doctor's order. They can be issued to you during or after your doctor's visit. A prescription, which is also denoted by the symbol "Rx," can be handwritten, faxed, electronically-transmitted, or telephoned in to the pharmacy by the doctor or doctor's agent.

Rules regulating prescribing and dispensing prescriptions are state-specific. Some of them, such as those for controlled substances, might also have restrictions concerning the mode of transmission, depending on state and federal laws. Patients often ask if they can fax or call in their own handwritten prescriptions. The answer? Absolutely *not*! Only a prescribing doctor or doctor's agent, such as a nurse, nurse practitioner or physician's assistant that is acting under the supervision of a doctor, can write or transmit prescriptions.

Quick Rx Tip: A patient cannot authorize or issue their own prescription. If you were issued a paper prescription, you are required to hand it to a pharmacist to be processed and dispensed.

A pharmacy cannot fill or prepare a brand-new prescription "ahead of time." When your prescription is received, the pharmacist can begin preparing it for you. (You can learn more about all the ways prescriptions can be sent to the pharmacy in Chapter 7.)

A doctor's prescription must have the following information:

- Patient information, including name, date of birth, and address.
- Medication information, including the name, strength, dose, quantity, and the date the prescription was issued.
- Doctor information, including name, phone, address, signature, and licensing information such as their Drug Enforcement Administration (DEA) number and/or their National Provider Identification (NPI) number.

The Drug Enforcement Administration (DEA) is the federal agency that regulates the distribution of controlled substances. The DEA number is a unique series of letters and numbers specific to the provider, authorizing them to prescribe controlled substances, and it can only be obtained by registering with the DEA. The

National Provider Identification (NPI) number is a series of 10 numbers assigned to a health care provider. It identifies the provider and is also needed for insurance billing purposes. The Centers for Medicare and Medicaid Services (CMS) requires all health care providers that bill for services to have an NPI number.

Over-the-Counter (OTC) Drugs

OTC products—including drugs, dietary vitamins, herbal supplements, and medical equipment—are available at the pharmacy and do not require a doctor's prescription. While they can play a significant role in patients' health, a trip to the pharmacy to pick up an OTC medicine can sometimes be daunting. Pharmacies can stock hundreds of over-the-counter products on their shelves, and there can be so many products and brands to choose from that it can get overwhelming.

To make things easier for yourself, locate designated aisles by using the overhead location markers and then carefully scan through the products for the drug that best matches your symptoms. It is a good idea to read the product package label carefully, paying close attention to the active and inactive ingredients, especially if you have drug allergies or sensitivities. If you take other medications, make sure that they are all compatible with each other so you don't end up with a bad reaction. If you are just plain clueless or need guidance—no worries! Go to the pharmacy counter and ask for a pharmacist consultation. When you speak with your pharmacist, describe the specific symptoms you are trying to treat. Let the pharmacist know how long you've had the symptoms and what products, if any, you have tried already.

For example, if you are trying to treat a cough, tell the pharmacist what type of cough it is. Is it a dry cough or a wet cough? A dry cough has no mucus, but a wet cough can produce mucous and phlegm.

Or, if you have a rash on your skin and you want to know what medicine you should use to help resolve it, the pharmacist might want to know what is causing you the most discomfort. Is the rash itchy? Is it irritated, discolored, or inflamed? Let the pharmacist know.

Based on the specific information you have provided, the pharmacist will make a recommendation that is available over-the-counter. Or they might refer you to see a doctor.

Quick Rx Tip: Before heading to the pharmacy, make your search easier by writing down the name of the product—especially if you are looking for a specific product. OTC products are often grouped together based on the symptoms they treat. Common OTC subgroups in a pharmacy are: First Aid, Stomach, Cold and Allergy, Pain, Dental, Ear, Eye and Nose, Vitamins, Sleep Aids, Skin Care and Medical Devices. For example if you are looking for an antibacterial product to put on a wound, look in the First Aid aisle. If you need an antacid for heartburn, you would look in the Stomach aisle.

Over-the-counter remedies are available for many conditions, such as:

- Topical fungal infections
- Yeast infections
- Urinary pain
- Skin conditions, including acne, psoriasis, eczema, lice, and diaper rash
- Wound care
- Allergic reactions/dermatitis from insect bites, poison ivy, and poison oak

- The common cold and flu
- Seasonal allergies
- Fever, pain, or migraine headaches
- Insomnia
- Smoking cessation
- Premenstrual syndrome
- Abdominal issues such as nausea, constipation, diarrhea, acid reflux, heartburn, and bloating
- Hemorrhoids
- Eye, ear, nose, and throat care
- Nutritional dietary supplement care

If you find yourself taking over-the-counter drugs for more than a week with no resolution of your symptoms, then you should consult with a doctor.

Behind-the-Counter (BTC) Products

Behind-the-counter products do not usually require a doctor's prescription but might be kept in the pharmacy behind the counter for legal reasons, storage requirements, or for safety reasons. They sometimes require identification to purchase them. Because certain types of BTC products are regulated by state or federal law, access to them can have limitations depending on the state you live in.

BTC products include cold, flu, sinus, and allergy medicines containing the active ingredient pseudoephedrine. Brand names include Sudafed, Mucinex-D, Advil Cold and Sinus, Aleve Cold and Sinus, Claritin-D, Allegra-D, Zyrtec-D, and their equivalent generic alternatives. The "D" in the product names refers to an ingredient that is used as a nasal decongestant—pseudoephedrine.

The sale of products that contain pseudoephedrine is regulated by state and federal law because they can be used illegally to manufacture the street drug "meth." Meth is a highly addictive synthetic stimulant that affects the central nervous system through the stimulation of dopamine receptors. At the height of the meth epidemic, meth dealers would obtain large amounts of pseudoephedrine products by posing as patients and purchasing them from the pharmacy. Meth use still continues to devastate people and their communities. It can have toxic long-term effects on the body, such as anorexia, tooth decay, skin deterioration, premature aging, and psychosis.

In an effort to prevent and curb meth abuse and diversion, identification requirements and quantity limits are mandatory in many states for products containing pseudoephedrine. Some states, including Oregon and Mississippi, have gone even further and require a doctors' prescription in order to dispense any products containing pseudoephedrine.

Quick Rx Tip: Many patients find these requirements a nuisance. It can be inconvenient that people can't stockpile cough and cold medicine when the product is on sale. But there's good reason for it. Your pharmacist is required to decline such a purchase.

Behind-the-counter products also include medicines that contain ephedrine, a compound that is similar to pseudoephedrine and is found in products like Bronkaid or Primatene tablets, which are used for the temporary relief of shortness of breath or asthma symptoms. They, too, have identification and purchase limit requirements.

Injectable needles and syringes are also kept behind the pharmacy counter. They are used to administer injectable medicines like insulin, fertility drugs, testosterone, and injectable supplements such as Vitamin B-12. Your ability to purchase behind-the-counter injectable syringes and needles without a prescription will vary from state to state. So check with the pharmacist for your state-specific requirements.

Injectable needles and syringes come in different lengths and sizes, so be sure you know the specifications for both the syringe and the needle that you need prior to arriving at the pharmacy. However, when in doubt, simply ask the pharmacist.

Choosing the Best Pharmacy for You

Choosing the right pharmacy for your medication needs is a personal decision that you should consider carefully. I recommend that you create a checklist of the top things you are looking for in a pharmacy. Then use the checklist to compare your options and make a decision. Here are some criteria to consider when selecting a pharmacy:

- If you have prescription insurance coverage, you want to select a pharmacy that is in your preferred network to get the lowest copayments and pricing on medications. Your prescription drugs might not be covered, or you might have to pay more if you use a pharmacy that is not in your insurance provider network.

- Location is an important factor to consider when choosing a pharmacy. Do you prefer a pharmacy that is close to your doctor's office? That way, you can pick up your medicines after your doctor's visit. Or would you prefer a location that is close to your home or work? Select a location that fits into your normal daily routine and is the easiest for you.

- Do you enjoy your interactions with the pharmacist and staff? Is the pharmacist knowledgeable and helpful? Whether you are a frequent flyer to the pharmacy or only go there every now and then, you want a pharmacist that cares and treats you with dignity and respect. Do you want a pharmacy that treats you like you are a prescription number, or do you want more? Place a high value on rapport and personal connections; they can make a world of difference in your pharmacy experience.

- Convenience is also something you might want to consider. Are you looking for just a standalone pharmacy where you can go in and out quickly and be on your way? Are you looking for the convenience of shopping for your groceries or household necessities while you wait for your prescriptions? Sometimes a one-stop-shop for all your needs might be your choice. Whatever you desire in a pharmacy, you can find a pharmacy that is tailored to meet those needs.

- The types of services offered by a pharmacy can also attract your loyalty. You will find that pharmacies provide an array of services—such as drug compounding, home delivery options, vaccinations, and onsite health care clinics—that can cater to your specific health needs.

Once you have selected a pharmacy, you should be consistent and use that pharmacy as your pharmacy home, which will give the pharmacist full access to your medication records. While dispensing your new prescription or refill, your pharmacist will check for adverse drug interactions between your current medications. If a medication you get at Pharmacy A interacts with a medicine you get at Pharmacy B, your pharmacist might not have access to that critical information if both pharmacies are not in the same network. This is why drugstore hopping can be unsafe.

For convenience, you can use a pharmacy that is part of a larger network or chain. Chain pharmacies typically have multiple locations, but they usually share an electronic database that makes communication and data sharing easier, thereby making it easier to detect potential safety interactions between medications. Except when there's an emergency, it is highly recommended to use the services of one pharmacy hub. There are so many pharmacies vying for your loyalty with offers of gift cards, free groceries, free medicines, discounted generic drugs, and other eye-popping promotions that it can be extremely tempting to start pharmacy hopping. But, in the long run, it is always safer to use one pharmacy as your pharmacy home.

The Patient-Pharmacy Challenge

Ask yourself this important question: How well do you know your pharmacy, its policies, processes, operations, and standard of practice? You might use the same pharmacy for years and still be clueless about the answers to those questions. The next time you visit the pharmacist, take this pharmacy challenge: talk to your pharmacist and complete the patient-pharmacy questionnaire on the next page. You'll find it will bridge the gaps in your understanding of your pharmacy, and the responses you get will help you better navigate your way around it.

Patient-Pharmacy Challenge Questionnaire:

Pharmacy name: ______________________________

Pharmacy phone: ______________________________

Pharmacy fax: ______________________________

Pharmacy address: ______________________________

Hours of operation: ______________________________

Name your pharmacist(s): ______________________________

Name your pharmacy technician(s): ______________________________

How long should I wait before going to the pharmacy to pick up my medication? ______________________________

How do I request a prescription refill? Do I contact the pharmacy or my doctor's office? ______________________________

____

Why do I sometimes get an incomplete or partial prescription order? ______________________________

____

If I get a partial order, when do I return to pick up the rest of my medication? ______________________________

How will I be notified when my medication is ready? __________

____

What other pharmacy services do you provide? __________

____

Do you take back medications for disposal? ________________

Can someone else pick up my medication for me? _____________

Do you have automatic medication refill services? How do I opt-in or opt-out of the program? ________________________________

____

What methods of payment do you accept? ________________

____

Can I make a payment over the phone? _____________________

Can I pick up my medication at a different location? Are there any restrictions? ____

____

How do I transfer my prescription to another pharmacy?

____

Can I return medications I don't need? ______________________

I don't have prescription insurance. How can I save on prescription drugs at your pharmacy? _______________________________

____

Do you have a pharmacy drive-through window? What products can I purchase through the drive-through? ________________

____

Now, take this opportunity to ask the pharmacist any miscellaneous questions that you've been curious about!

____

Knowledge Checkpoint

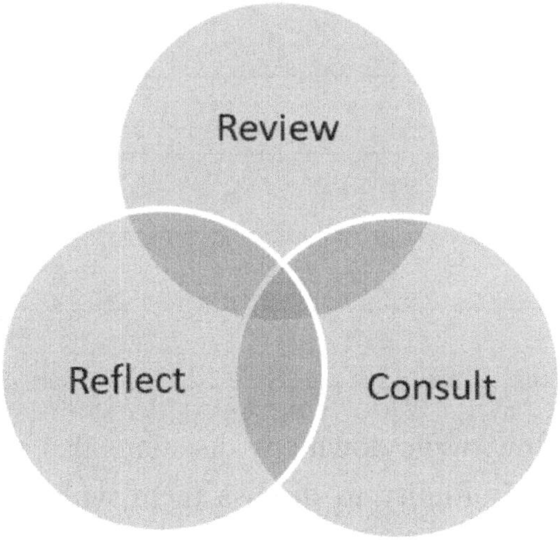

REVIEW: In the preceding three chapters, you learned the importance of knowing the names of the medications you take and of having an up-to-date medication list. You discovered some hidden clues that could help you better understand your medications. You also took a closer look into a typical day in the life of a community pharmacist. Finally, you reviewed some criteria to consider when choosing the best pharmacy for your health care needs.

REFLECT: Take a moment to reflect on what you have learned and then answer these questions: Do you know the names of all your routine medications? Do you have an up-to-date medication list? If you do not, then take a moment to make one now and be sure it contains the names, dosage, use and prescribing doctor's information for all the medications you take.

CONSULT: Now, write down any questions that you have. Then, take the next opportunity to discuss them with your health care provider and get the answers you need.

Chapter 7
Getting Comfortable with Prescriptions

The Anatomy of a Prescription

The pharmacist receives prescription orders from doctors throughout the day and processes them as soon as they are received. They can receive prescriptions in several ways, including:

- Paper. Your doctor physically hands you a paper copy or written prescription, and you take that to the pharmacist.
- Fax. Your doctor faxes your prescription directly to the pharmacy. A faxed prescription is only valid when it comes directly from the prescribing doctor. By law, a pharmacist cannot accept a faxed prescription from a patient.
- Verbal. Your doctor or doctor's agent calls your prescription into the pharmacy by phone. The doctor can call in a telephone order to a designated prescriber's voicemail or speak directly to the pharmacist.
- Electronically. Your doctor can send an electronic prescription to the pharmacy through an electronic portal. Because of variability in workload and connectivity, electronic prescriptions can sometimes have a lag time before the pharmacy receives them.
- Transfer. Sometimes an existing eligible prescription can be transferred from one pharmacy to another.

The Review Process

When a pharmacist receives a medication order, it goes through several levels of review before it can be dispensed to you. Your pharmacist:

- reviews the prescription for validity, accuracy, completeness, and dose appropriateness.
- reviews patient medication and health history to check for patient-specific contraindications, allergies, or drug-to-drug interactions.
- reviews the prescription data entry to ensure you get correct and easy-to-understand instructions with your medication.
- prepares your medication by counting and measuring the specific quantity, transferring it into the appropriate pill bottle or container, and attaching patient-specific labeling.
- performs a quality-assurance check by physically inspecting your pill bottle or package and providing you with a detailed drug information literature.
- packages your prescription and places it in the designated pick-up area, so it is ready for you to pick up.

If, during the review process, your pharmacist notices that a prescription is incomplete or identifies any major allergies or drug interactions, your order will end up being delayed. It will be placed on hold, requiring consultation with your doctor first. The pharmacist will attempt to contact your doctor to inform them about the issues or irregularities and, if needed, replace the medication with a safer one. The pharmacist cannot make any changes to the prescription without the consent of the doctor. Of course, this can be frustrating because you want to start taking your medication as quickly as possible so you can feel better. But the pharmacist is required to follow protocol and cannot make any changes based on what you tell them.

In fact, a prescription is a legal, medical document, and the pharmacist is required by law to obtain verification directly from the doctor who wrote it. Only after your doctor gives legal consent to the pharmacist can any necessary changes or alterations be made to complete your medication order.

While most doctors try to respond to a pharmacist's request as quickly as possible, they are also often quite busy and might not be available to respond immediately. The pharmacist sometimes has to leave a message or send a fax request and wait for a response.

There are some things you can do as a patient to help you get your medication as quickly as possible, including:

- Report all drug allergies you have to the pharmacist. Every prescription you get will be screened against your drug allergies to ensure you always receive medications that are safe.

- Make sure the pharmacy has your current mailing address and phone number. The pharmacist might need to contact you about a delay or an issue with your prescription.

- Bring your insurance card along with your prescription. Having the physical or electronic copy of your insurance card will always save you time at the pharmacy. It can mean the difference between your prescription taking a few minutes to complete or taking much longer.

- Call ahead before you pick up your prescription to ensure your medicines are ready for you. Many pharmacies can notify you by phone, email or text that they're ready, so inquire about the types of notification services your pharmacy offers. When you do get a notification, don't assume your order is ready unless the message specifically says so. Listen to or read the entire message. Your pharmacy might be notifying you of an issue with your order.

- Always verify patient-specific information such as your full name and date of birth when communicating with your pharmacy. Don't be offended when the pharmacist asks you to verify personal information during these interactions. They do so for your safety. Patients often have similar names and dates of birth, and parents and children sometimes have similar names, too. For example, sons and fathers might have the same name, with a Junior or Senior suffix. It is always important that you verify this information to help prevent medication errors.

- Don't forget your ID. Prescriptions for some medications, such as controlled substances and products containing pseudoephedrine, require you to show identification for purchase. Don't be offended when asked to do so; it is simply a legal requirement.

- We all have nicknames that we might prefer to be called. To prevent confusion, use the same name at the doctor's office and the pharmacy. That way, there won't be added confusion or delays to your order. For example, consider that a pharmacist receives an electronic medication order for patient Patricia Johnson. But before the pharmacist starts to process the order, a database search is done to see if Patricia Johnson has an existing account with the pharmacy. If an exact match isn't found, a new patient account will be created for Patricia's order. A few days later, when a patient comes to pick up her medications, she gives the name Tracey Lamar at the pick-up counter. The pharmacist does an extensive search, but she finds no prescription available under that name. After further inquiry, the patient reveals that her legal name is Patricia Johnson, but her nickname is Tracey, and her maiden name is Lamar. After time spent on further verification, she is able to pick up her medication. However, the simple pick-up process took much longer than it had to because the new account had to be reconciled and corrected.

Quick Rx Tip: Before picking up your medicine, check with the pharmacy to confirm the status of your prescription; don't assume your medication is ready. Most pharmacies have digital platforms, such as text messaging, phone apps, and email alerts, that can be useful tools to help you stay informed about your prescriptions.

Your Prescription Order

To prevent delays in the ordering of your prescription, it is important that your doctor issue you a complete prescription that contains all the information that the pharmacist will need to properly prepare and dispense your medicine. If the doctor issues you a paper prescription, it must be written on tamper-resistant paper. Doing so is an industry standard because the paper has security features that allow the pharmacist to validate the authenticity of the prescription. All prescriptions must contain:

1. Doctor's name, office address, phone number, and fax number (if available)
2. Doctor's National Provider Identification (NPI) number or Drug Enforcement Administration (DEA) number, if prescribing a controlled substance
3. The date the prescription was written

4. Patient identifier: name, date of birth or age, address
5. Medication name, strength or concentration, and dose
6. Medication quantity
7. Specific instructions for use
8. Number of refills allowed
9. Notice if generic substitution is permitted or if the brand name is medically necessary
10. Doctor's signature

It is now common practice for medical facilities to give nurse practitioners and physician assistants authority to prescribe medications. When that happens, the supervising doctor's credentials must also be provided on the prescription to comply with state and federal prescribing laws and insurance plan requirements.

It is always a good idea to review your prescription hardcopy before you leave the office to ensure that all of the required information is on your paper prescription. It is also a good idea to know exactly what your doctor is giving you. Engage the doctor before leaving the office so that you clearly understand what medicines are being issued to you.

Sample prescription formats

RX

Name of Doctor/Clinic/Hospital

Address, phone, and fax number

NPI and DEA number (if applicable)

Date RX written

Patient name, address, date of birth

Drug name, strength, quantity, and directions for use

Number of refills allowed

Generic substitution allowed? Brand medically necessary?

Provider's name and signature

Include Supervising Doctor's full name and information (NPI and DEA is applicable) when provider is a Physician Assistant or Nurse Practitioner.

Test your Knowledge!

Now, test your knowledge! Here are some prescription samples. Can you identify any potential issues or omissions?

RX Jane Doe, MD. NPI 1010101010

123 Hospital Blvd. Any town, U.S.A. 123-145-7890

5/19/Year

John Doe 6 Joys Blvd. Any town U.S.A DOB: 1/1/75

Rx: Amoxicillin 500mg tablet #30

1 tablet by mouth 3 times per day

Refills: 0

Generic substitution is permitted

Jane Doe

(Rx 1)

The prescription (Rx 1) has no issues.

RX Jane Doe, MD. NPI 1010101010

123 Hospital Blvd. Any town, U.S.A. 123-145-7890

2/28/Year

John Doe 6 Joys Blvd. Any town U.S.A DOB: 1/1/75

Diazepam 5mg #2. Refills: 0

1 tablet by mouth night before procedure and 1 tablet 1 hour before procedure

Generic substitution is permitted

Jane Doe

(Rx 2)

The prescription (Rx 2) is missing a DEA number. Diazepam is a controlled substance, and the ordering physician's DEA number is required on the prescription.

RX Jane Doe, MD. NPI 1010101010

123 Hospital Blvd. Any town, U.S.A. 123-145-7890

John Doe 6 Joys Blvd. Any Town U.S.A DOB: 1/1/75

Prednisone 20mg #9.

2 tablets by mouth daily for 3 days, then 1 tablet daily for 3 days

Refills: 0

Generic substitution is permitted

Jane Doe

(Rx 3)

The prescription (Rx 3) is missing the written date. A prescription must contain the original date issued.

RX Jane Doe, MD. NPI 1010101010

123 Hospital Blvd. Any town, U.S.A. 123-145-7890

11/15/Year

John Doe 6 Joys Blvd. Any town U.S.A DOB: 1/1/16

Cephalexin 250mg/5ml Suspension #1bottle

5ml by mouth twice daily

Refills: 0

Generic substitution is permitted

Jane Doe

(Rx 4)

The prescription above is missing the specific quantity to dispense. For liquid medications, the quantity prescribed should be designated in milliliters or fluid ounces. Liquid medicines come in different manufacturer stock bottles and sizes, so accuracy matters. The exact quantity in milliliters or fluid ounces is needed to calculate and dispense the quantity sufficient for the duration of therapy. It is also needed to accurately bill the insurance plan for the prescribed medication.

RX Jane Doe, MD. NPI 1010101010

123 Hospital Blvd. Any town, U.S.A. 123-145-7890

9/18//Year

John Doe 6 Joys Blvd. Any Town U.S.A DOB: 1/1/75

Albuterol 90 mcg inhaler # 1 tube

Use as directed. Refills: 5

Generic substitution is permitted

Jane Doe

(Rx 5)

The prescription (Rx 5) is missing the patient's directions for use. It is not clear how the patient is to take the medicine. Although the doctor might have told the patient how to use it at their visit, patients often forget. In practice, "Use as Directed" prescription instructions are highly discouraged and should be limited to medications that are available in prepackaged dose packs only. Dose packs are made with pre-printed manufacturer instructions on the package, which allows the patient to simply follow the instructions on the package.

For all other medications, specific instructions on the prescription are needed so that the patient can take it correctly, to ensure that the patient is counseled accurately, and to bill the insurance plan correctly. It also protects against unintentional medication errors.

Pursuant to federal and state laws, an incomplete prescription is considered invalid. As a result, it is common for insurance plans to reduce or cancel payments to pharmacies for dispensed medications—already in the hands of the patient—due to an incomplete prescription. It can ultimately cost a pharmacy thousands of dollars in revenue and, over time, deal a serious blow to a pharmacy's bottom line. These "chargebacks" can occur for many reasons:

- The quantity prescribed by the doctor and dispensed by the pharmacist exceeds what the insurance plan will pay for.
- The days of supply or duration of therapy exceed what the insurance plan will pay for.
- The prescription from the doctor is incomplete or contains omissions. Examples include no signature, corrections are not initialed, no written date, or no DEA number on controlled medicines.
- The hardcopy (paper) prescription was not written on tamper-resistant prescription paper.
- The prescription, written by a physician's assistant or nurse practitioner, does not include the name of the supervising doctor and prescribing information.

Quick Rx Tip: What is a prescription chargeback? When the pharmacist dispenses a medication to a patient with insurance coverage, the insurance plan reimburses the pharmacy for the cost of providing the medication. A chargeback occurs when the insurance plan essentially rescinds payment, taking a portion or all of the reimbursed money back from the pharmacy.

When a pharmacist receives an order for a prescription that doesn't have all of the necessary medication information, they are required to get clarification from the prescribing doctor. For the patient and doctor, the calls from the pharmacist might seem trivial or unnecessary, but it is the mandatory duty and responsibility of the professional. Not doing so could result in costly fines, chargebacks, and sanctions on the part of both the pharmacy and pharmacist.

Decoding the Prescription

Decoding a doctor's prescription, especially a handwritten paper copy, is an art and a science! Many doctors still use handwritten paper prescriptions, and quite a few prescribers still use roman numerals on prescriptions. On occasion, I have to dust off my reference guide to decipher an order! Let's be honest, have you ever tried reading your doctor's handwritten prescription? It really makes for a good brain exercise. Patients are frequently amazed at my ability to make out what seems to be a blatantly unreadable prescription.

Doctors write prescriptions using standardized nomenclature, referred to as "sig codes," which enable the pharmacist to read the prescription. From a pharmacist's perspective, it is also part training and skill. Pharmacists often interact with prescribers frequently enough that, eventually, they come to learn the unique characteristics of their prescriptions, writing, and penmanship, and deciphering becomes second nature. Nevertheless, I have been stumped clueless many times, too, when I couldn't easily make out a prescription. When that occurs, the prescriber is only a phone call away to help clarify the order.

With the expansion of electronic medical records technology, more and more prescribers are using print format hard copies and electronic orders instead of manually handwriting prescriptions. This allows for better clarity and accuracy. The pharmacist will transcribe and translate your doctor's prescription into simple and easy-to-understand instructions for you to follow.

It is very important that you review your medicine bottle before beginning your medicine. It might sound trivial, but patients often call, in a panic, because they assumed they knew how to take their medications but subsequently took the wrong dose without even reading the label on the bottle.

Quick Rx Tip: Do not make any assumptions when drugs are involved. When you prepare to take your medication:

- STOP and review the label on your pill bottle
- STOP and review the enclosed drug information package
- STOP and review the contents of your pill bottle

The Label on the Bottle

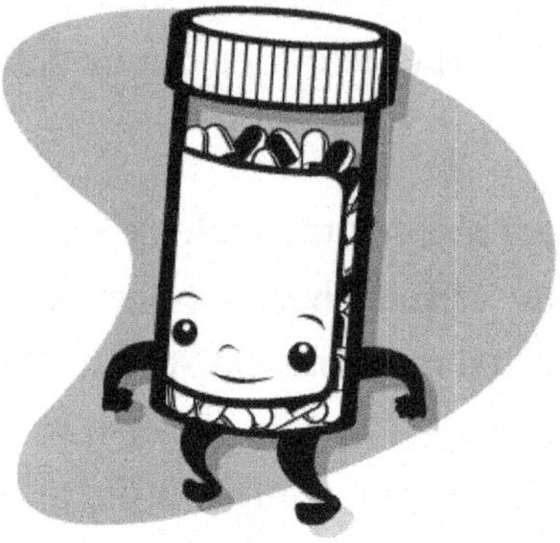

Jane Doe — Date: May 4, 2021

Patient Address

RX#: 100001

Zolpidem 10mg Tablets #30

(Name of drug manufacturer & physical description)

Take 1 tablet at bedtime as needed for sleep. Use sparingly.

1 Refill before November 4

Dr. Six Joys

Caution: May cause sedation. Do not drive or operate machinery. Keep away from children.

Sunnyside pharmacy, Address and Phone Number

Like your prescription, the label on your prescription bottle contains important information about your medicine. The label must include:

- The patient's name and address
- The name, strength, dose, and quantity of medication
- The name of the drug manufacturer and the physical description, if applicable
- Dosage: how to take the medication, and how many times a day to take it
- Special precautions or warnings about the medication. For example: it requires refrigeration; take with food; do not drive; swallow whole; do not crush; apply topically; might cause sedation; shake well.
- The date the prescription was filled
- The prescription number to reference for refills or questions
- The number of refills approved by the prescribing physician. A refill means your doctor has authorized you to get another order in the future when it becomes due.

- The name of the doctor prescribing the medicine.
- The dispensing pharmacy's name, address, and contact information.

Quick Rx Tip: The prescription number on the label of your pill bottle is a computer-generated series of numbers that is assigned to a prescription order. The number can change; do not get upset if it does. Your pharmacist has no control over it.

Physicians sometimes send new prescription orders even if the patient still has active refills on their existing medicine. The pharmacist cannot combine the refills together because such orders can have different parameters, such as the original authorized date and the quantity. When this happens, the pharmacy will typically place the duplicate prescription on hold for the patient until they use up their refills from the previous order.

Quick Rx Tip: If your old bottle says that there are no refills left, don't panic or frantically call the doctor's office. Check with your pharmacy first to see if you have any other available refills on file. It is very common to have medicines under different prescription numbers.

If you have refills on a non-controlled medicine, they are typically valid for up to a year from the date the original prescription was written; however, it will depend on the state it was written in, since pharmacy laws can vary from state to state. Refill allocation is determined by the doctor. The prescribing doctor has the ultimate authority to adjust the refill parameters of the prescription. When you run out of refills, you can ask the pharmacist to contact your prescribing doctor to obtain additional refills. However, the pharmacist cannot dictate to your physician the number of refills to provide to you. Don't get upset when your doctor only authorized one refill when you expected more.

Refills for a controlled medicine are generally good for up to six months from the original written date of the prescription unless your doctor or specific state law dictates otherwise.

By law, Class 2 prescriptions for controlled substances will allow no refills. They contain the highest class of controlled substance allowed for medical use. The doctor should write you a new prescription order each time you need one.

Your bottle's label should show the date your refills will expire. If you don't refill your medicine before the expiration date, the refills expire and become void. A new prescription from your doctor will be needed to renew it.

Here are some examples:

- Your doctor wrote you a prescription for an Albuterol inhaler on a certain date. He gave you 12 refills, which means the prescription is good for one year if you refill it on a monthly basics. Your prescription will expire the following year on the same date.

- Your doctor gave you a prescription for Premarin tablets with two refills. That means you can get the medicine up to three times—the first time plus two more refills after that. After you use up all of your refills, there is no more left on your order, and refill approval from your doctor will be needed. If you don't use all your refills, the prescription will still expire the following year on the same date.

- Your doctor gave you a prescription for Tramadol tablets with zero refills. After you use up your medicine, there is no refill available, and a doctors' approval will be needed for more medicine.

Let's practice reading a prescription bottle. What does this prescription bottle tell you?

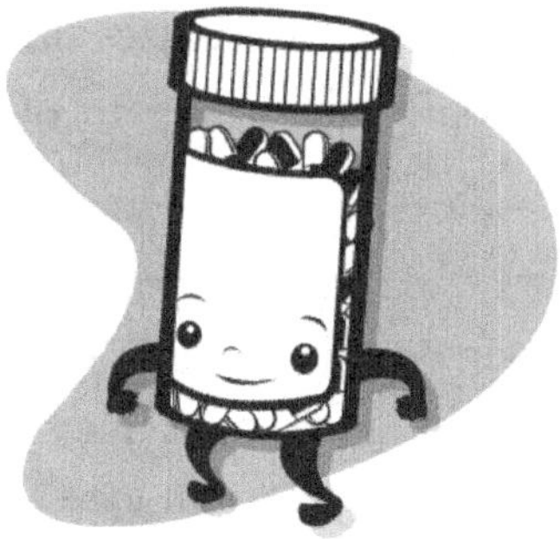

Jane Doe **January 1, 2021**

Patient address

RX#: 123456

Ciprofloxacin 500mg Tablets #20

(White oval shaped, Apotec manufacturer)

Take 1 tablet by mouth twice daily for 10 days.

0 Refill from Dr Six Joys

Take until all finished. Keep away from children. Take with food. May cause nausea.

Sunnyside pharmacy, Address and Phone number

The medication Ciprofloxacin is an antibiotic used to treat bacterial infections. The patient follows the specific instructions on the bottle by taking one tablet orally two times a day, morning and evening, until they finish the entire supply of medicine. The patient should not take the medicine on an empty stomach, as it might cause nausea or an upset stomach.

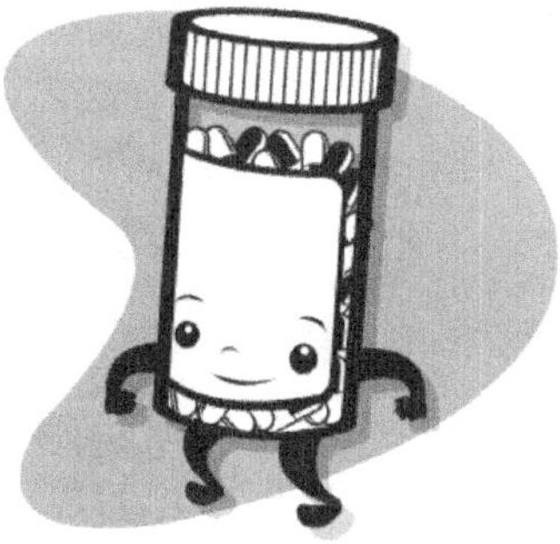

Jane Doe **March 17, 2021**

Patient Address

RX#: 56789

Ethinyl estradiol/norethindrone acetate FE 1/20 MCG Tablet #28

(White round, Actavis manufacturer)

Take 1 tablet orally same time every day.

12 Refills Until March16 following year.

Dr. Six Joys

May cause nausea. Take with food. Keep away from children.

Sunnyside pharmacy, Address and Phone number

Ethinyl estradiol/norethindrone acetate is an oral contraceptive (birth control) medicine containing estrogen and progestin hormones. It is taken orally once daily, preferably at a consistent time. This medication might cause nausea, so it can be taken with food. Patients have been known to incorrectly assume that birth control pills are taken only on days that intercourse occurs. This is not the case. Unlike emergency contraceptives that are specifically used up to 72 hours after intercourse, regular, daily-use oral contraceptives should consistently be taken daily according to the medicine's instructions.

Quick Rx Tip: Always follow your doctor's orders by using the instructions that comes with your medicine. When in doubt, STOP and contact your pharmacist or health care provider.

Decoding Your Doctor's Instructions

Since your medicine bottle label includes instructions about how your doctor wants you to take it, be sure to review them carefully before you begin taking your medicine. If you have any questions about taking your medicine, or if you find the instructions unclear, call the pharmacy and get your questions answered. When in doubt, call the pharmacist to check it out.

Here are some helpful explanations:

Instructions	**Example**
As needed	Take your medicine only when you need it. For example, if your label says, "Ondansetron 4mg. Take 1 tablet every 8 hours as needed for nausea," only take the medicine if you feel nauseated. You can repeat the dose in eight hours if you need to.
Inhale into lungs	Place the mouthpiece of the inhaler in the mouth, making sure to have a good seal. Depress inhaler, inhale deeply, and hold the breath for a few seconds to allow the medicine to reach the lungs.
Intramuscularly	Inject drug into the muscle.
Keep refrigerated	The medicine is best stored in the refrigerator. Many drugs, including insulin and some reconstituted antibiotics, require refrigeration.
Once daily	Take only one time a day. For example, if your label says to take two tablets once daily, it means to take two tablets at the same time once every day.
Rectally	Unwrap and insert into the rectum.
Spray into nostril	The medicine should be sprayed into the nose.
STAT	Take immediately or as soon as possible.
Subcutaneously	Inject drug into the subcutaneous

	tissue under the skin.
Sublingually	Place medicine under the tongue and allow to dissolve.
Take every day or take daily	For example, if the label says: "Losartan 50mg. Take one tablet every day," take one tablet once a day.
Take four times a day	Take your medicine four times per day, typically every six hours.
Take monthly	Take once a month, approximately every 28 to 30 days.
Take three times a day	For example, if the label says "Hydroxyzine 25mg. Take 1 tablet 3 times a day," take one tablet each in the morning, afternoon, and night.
Take till all gone	This instruction means to take your medicine as instructed until the bottle is empty. For example, if your label says, "Amoxicillin 500mg #30. Take one capsule 3 times a day until all taken," then complete the entire course of therapy until all the medicine is finished. In this example, that would occur in ten days.
Take twice a day	For example, if the label says "Penicillin 500mg. Take one tablet twice a day," take one tablet two times each day, such as morning and evening.
Take twice a week	Take two times a week, such as Monday and Thursday.

Take weekly	Take once a week or every seven days
Topically	Apply the drug externally, directly onto the skin. Topical medications include patches, creams, solutions, ointments, and gels.
Use as directed	Follow the directions from the manufacturer found on the package or the specific instructions your doctor gave you. Medications that come in a “dose pack” will have prepackaged instructions, so be sure to read those. Examples of medicines that come in dose packs are Azithromycin, Methylprednisolone, and Prednisone.

Some medications come in liquid formulations. Here are some helpful conversions to be aware of:

Liquid Measurement Equivalencies

- 1 teaspoon = 5ml = 5cc
- 1/2 teaspoon = 2.5ml = 2.5cc
- 3/4 teaspoon = 3.75ml = 3.75cc
- 1 ½ teaspoon = 7.5ml = 7.5cc
- 2 teaspoons = 10ml = 10cc
- 1 tablespoon = 15ml = 15cc
- 1 ounce = 30ml = 30cc

Quick Rx Tip: When measuring the dose of liquid medicines, use the measuring syringe or spoon provided by the pharmacist. Household utensils may not accurately measure the dose needed. If you ever need a medication dosing syringe or spoon, ask the pharmacist.

Your Prescription Insurance

If you have prescription insurance, you should review your prescription insurance information package when it arrives, as boring as it might be to read. Do not assume that your prescription plan is the same as it was the previous year. Keep the information in a memorable, accessible place for future reference. It's important that you understand the details of your prescription insurance plan and know what to expect when things happen. Know what your copayment, deductible, and coinsurance amounts are. Get to know your preferred provider network and what services, providers, and/or pharmacies are covered under your plan.

Many pharmacy benefit providers are using "preferred pharmacy networks," where you can only fill your prescriptions at a pharmacy that is in the network. If you use an out-of-network pharmacy, your insurance company might deny your order or give your medicines a much higher price tag.

When you receive new prescription insurance cards, discard the old ones and place your new cards in your wallet immediately. Prescription insurance cards might not always have dates on them, which is why you want to discard those that are old or expired as soon as you receive updated ones. Presenting an expired prescription card to the pharmacist will almost always cause needless delays. Also, ensure that your covered dependents—your spouse or children—get a copy of your new insurance card, too.

If you have prescription insurance and your doctor starts you on a medication that you expect to be on for a while, find out if you are eligible to get a larger supply, three months' worth, for example. If so, find out if you are eligible to get it from your retail pharmacy. Or does your insurance plan require you to use their mail-order pharmacy? These are important questions that you should pay close attention to when reviewing your benefits package.

Insurance benefits packages often include:

- **A summary of your coverage.** What you have or don't have, including medical, pharmacy, vision, and dental. The summary might also provide dollar amounts on annual deductible, coinsurance, out-of-pocket limits, and copayments.
- **Detailed information about coverage.** Details about health services or medications that are covered and those that are not covered under your plan.
- **How to find an in-network health care provider.** Not all doctors or pharmacies are covered. Some insurance companies have a preferred network of providers. Educate yourself on the details of your plan and call your insurance company if you have any questions.
- **Who to contact if you have questions regarding eligibility or coverage.** If your insurance is through your employer, you might need to contact your Human Resources Benefits department or your insurance plan directly.

- **How to change or update your personal information.** It is important that your insurance company has updated information about you to ensure that your prescription claims are processed accurately. Inaccurate information such as incorrect address or birth date might cause delayed or rejected claims at the pharmacy. Patients often have nicknames or preferred names. Ensure that the name you use at your provider and pharmacy matches the name on your insurance card.
- **Who to contact for life status changes.** These might include name change due to marriage or divorce and new dependents due to marriage, birth, or adoption.
- **Additional benefits and services.** Find out what else you might be interested in, including prescription mail order, telephone health advice line, telemedicine, and smoking cessation programs.
- **Copayment Tier and Access Information.** Information about their prescription copayment tier structure as well as information about how to access your pharmacy plan preferred formulary medication list. This can help you better understand the cost of your medications.

Chapter 8
Sticker Shock

People are increasingly getting sticker shock at the pharmacy counter! And rightfully so, because medications costs are eating into the household budget of many Americans. Prescription costs rank third among Americans' health care expenses.[13] Americans pay 50% more for similar drug products compared to other countries.[14] With such high-priced health care, one would think that we are healthier compared to other Western countries that spend less, but it's not so! The U.S. ranks last in health outcomes when compared to Australia, Canada, France, Germany, Netherlands, New Zealand, Norway, Sweden, Switzerland, and the United Kingdom.[15] By far, the most common questions that patients have are about medication costs.

There are many reasons for the growing cost of health care and medicines. Here are my observations from my experience as a pharmacist.

Health Literacy

When people lack proficiency with health-related issues, it can result in making poor choices about their care, which can lead to unnecessary and costly spending. *Health literacy* is the ability to understand and use health information correctly; it plays an important role in our ability to make informed health care decisions for ourselves. There is no doubt that barriers exist, such as language, education, and age, that can make it challenging to process health information. As much as health care providers try to accommodate barriers when they are caring for their patients, if you recognize the barriers that you have and seek available resources, it will help you make better health decisions.

For example, if you have a language barrier, bring someone to accompany you to the pharmacy or doctor's office who can help translate, coordinate, and process health information. For the elderly, designating a caretaker to assist in decision-making is important. When my mother had eye surgery, as her primary caretaker, I was present for all of her pre- and post-surgical appointments as well as during the surgery. I was there to coordinate her care and to ensure that all the right questions were asked and answered.

A study was conducted to directly measure health literacy in adults. According to the Agency for Healthcare Research and Quality, close to 80 million adults do not have adequate health literacy. They defined "health literacy" to include:[16]

- the ability to understand medication instructions, diagnosis, and treatment as well as how to complete health information documents.
- knowledge of self-management of illness and general concepts about maintaining good health
- an understanding of how health insurance works

In the study, adult health literacy was measured on a scale of 0 to 500, with points determined as follows:

- Below basic health literacy: 0 to 184 points
- Basic health literacy: 185 to 225 points

- Intermediate health literacy: 226 to 309 points
- Proficient health literacy: 310 to 500 points

Below are some results of the study:

- 14% below basic health literacy
- 22% basic health literacy
- 53% intermediate health literacy
- 12% proficient health literacy

If the goal is for most people to be proficient in health literacy—and it should be—then having 12% adult proficiency shows there is a lot of work to be done to get there. In the meantime, there are many routine health care encounters and choices that patients face every day, including:

- Completing documents, such as medical and prescription histories. Question: *Do you know the names and dosages of the medicines you take?*
- Deciding which procedures or services to choose from when presented with options.
- Reviewing insurance documents, such as benefits information. Question: *Do you know what a deductible is? What is your yearly health care deductible? Do you know what a preferred provider is?*
- Choosing the right insurance plan for you when presented with several options.
- Choosing between similar over-the-counter products.
- Reading prescription information and understanding how to take your medicine.
- Deciding between self-management and going to the doctor.

- Deciding whether to purchase that miracle drug you heard about on the radio?

Now, ask yourself: *Am I able to complete these tasks?* What grade would you give yourself on your health literacy? How would you rate yourself? Are you proficient enough? Are you confident that you are making the right health care choices? If you have any doubt about your ability to perform these tasks, then you've got work to do.

In today's health care system, it is an absolute necessity to be an informed patient:

An informed patient understands that they, too, have a role to play in keeping the cost of their health care down.

An informed patient uses information to empower and to decide which services to use.

An informed patient asks questions.

An informed patient understands that the choices they make drive the market.

An informed patient understands that the health care industry is a business.

An informed patient knows how to make the system work to meet their needs.

An informed patient clearly communicates with their health care provider and uses each medical encounter as an opportunity to expand their health literacy.

Consumer Culture

Another factor that contributes to the high cost of care is consumerism; American consumer culture is alive and well and affects how we use health care services. The culture that "more is better" applies to health care, as well. The system that encourages overconsumption does not coach patients adequately about how to be better consumers. The reality is that we live in a capitalist economy, and although the health care code of our medical professionals is "Do no harm," it is not the same for our health care system.

Unfortunately, in our society, money is king—even when it comes to health care. Health care in American has evolved into a transactional engagement that often places a higher value on profit and sales than on patient care. While ensuring access to health care is important, we need to also focus on educating consumers so that when they access care, they make better choices and are able to navigate the system with less confusion and frustration. With the passage of The Health Care Affordability Act, more Americans are able to purchase health insurance and have access to health care services. With the new influx of consumers, more emphasis is needed on patient health education and awareness.

I find that many patients are clueless about critical aspects of their care. They fall prey to deceptive advertising, products, and services that take advantage of the consumer-culture hype. For example, patients often come to the pharmacy in search of "As Seen on TV" products with miracle cures, and they are ready to purchase products without having any basic knowledge about them and without having done any research on what the products contain. Some believe that the chain of care and their role in it consists of: I get sick, I go see a doctor, he gives me a pill, I take the pill, and then I get well.

Consumer culture has become more prevalent in our health care system as more hospitals, clinics, and doctors use ads to reach consumers. Ads promise the latest technology in treating and diagnosing diseases. One ad for a local hospital, for example, promotes the facility as "the cure for the common hospital." There are ads that target men with erectile dysfunction, promising cheap innovating therapy that will cure them completely. And yes, there are numerous street signs for pain management clinics promising to completely rid patients of their pain. There are ads for skincare products that claim to reverse aging and ads for supplements that claim to suck up all your fat and make your body look picture-perfect. There are ads for vitamins for your ears, eyes, legs, stomach, brain, bones—virtually every part of the body.

Health care in the U.S. today feels like a commodity for sale. Consumerism in the health care industry has led to overconsumption and waste, and patients are naïve to the real costs. The push to get patients a large 90-day medicine supply on all their medications sounds great. But what happens when therapy is changed or discontinued and you are stuck with a stockpile of medications that you no longer need? There is a lot of waste. Yet, unfortunately, you can't walk into your pharmacy and say, "Oh, by the way, I don't need the rest of my medicine anymore, and I expect to return them for a refund." Once you purchase your prescription medicines, you are stuck with them and cannot return them simply because of buyer's remorse.

In a medication take-back event, the DEA collected over 200 tons of unused medicine from patients across the nation in one single day.[17] Two hundred tons! That is the weight of a blue whale, the largest animal in the world.

Defensive Medicine

Defensive medicine is another contributing factor in the high cost of health care in America. Defensive medicine occurs when a health care provider bases treatment decisions for their patients primarily on the intention to limit exposure to malpractice litigation instead of what is in the best interest of the patient. The practice of defensive medicine is a real occurrence in health care today, and it adds up to $45 billion per year.[18] The practice is blamed on a lack of medical tort reform and the liability claims against doctors. It causes health care professionals to increase the use of diagnostic tests, procedures, and medicines that might be unnecessary but prove due diligence and protect against liability lawsuits. Debate is still going on regarding how to effectively manage defensive medicine. We cannot simply legislate defensive medicine away since it has become the status quo. As providers of care, we have to recognize the bias we bring to our profession and work within our circle of influence to change those practices. We have to recognize that all the decisions we make as providers directly impact patients and their health care costs. Since many of the choices medical professionals make directly dictate what services patients use, it is also our responsibility to ensure we keep costs in mind when making decisions. Instead of going with the most expensive procedure or medicine, we should choose less-costly options that can deliver comparable results.

Signs of defensive medicine practices can be seen in:

- overuse of antibiotics
- overuse of Caesarian section deliveries
- the unnecessary repetition of or unnecessary ordering of labs and diagnostic tests
- overprescribing of medications

As a patient, do not be passive in your care. Engage in proactive discussions with your health care provider about the specifics of your care. Make sure you understand why certain tests, procedures, or medications are being ordered or recommended. Be your own advocate and an active participant in your health care decisions.

Direct-to-Consumer Advertising of Prescription Drugs

In health care, direct-to-consumer advertising is big business. It often leads to consumers seeking specific drugs from doctors regardless of whether the drug is right for them. But patients often don't realize that the cost of drug marketing and sales is passed on to the consumer. In one year alone, U.S. drug companies can spend up to $40 billion on sales and marketing.[19] All of us have heard, seen, or read a prescription drug ad. They can be funny, scary, and sometimes shocking. They can tear at your heartstrings or make you sad or happy. They'll depict someone playing golf, or at a picnic, or in the bathtub, and we begin to picture ourselves doing those things. The ad might begin by saying that a drug can help you with a particular condition; it might depict a person whose mood changes from sad to happy after starting the medicine. Or they'll show someone who takes a particular drug and now is the life of the party.

Animated television drug ads are becoming more common and often appeal to viewers because of the humor and seemingly non-threatening disposition. You almost forget that you are watching an ad for a prescription drug. Such ads definitely get an A+ for creativity, but they come at a cost to patients.

Drug companies want their ads to play on your emotions and naiveté so that you feel motivated to see your doctor and inquire about their brand of medication. Their catchy ads help increase their name recognition; people are more likely to remember the name of a drug when it's in a catchy ad. But these catchy ads don't mention the fact that the drugs are brand-name drugs and there might be generic alternatives available on the market that would provide a similar effect but cost a lot less. The drug manufacturers provide coupons in their ads, too, further motivating people to ask their doctors about the drug without recognizing that there are other cost-effective therapeutic options available.

Before 1985, U.S. drug companies were not allowed to market prescription drugs directly to consumers; the U.S. and New Zealand are now the only countries in the world where direct-to-consumer prescription drug ads are legal.[20]

Our culture of direct-to-consumer drug ads can cause overuse of medicines because patients often try to self-diagnose their symptoms and act as their own doctor. It can also be a nuisance for physicians who find themselves torn between prescribing a drug a patient is specifically requesting versus doing what is best for the patient. In fact, in order to keep patients happy, some health care providers sometimes give in and give patients what they want.

The bottom line is that you should not start taking any medication simply because you saw an ad for it. When you start making demands to your doctor to prescribe a medication you saw on TV or heard about on the radio, then you are feeding into the negative cycle of defensive medicine. Trust that your health care provider will make recommendations suited to your needs.

It's important not to treat medications like a new, exclusive, and expensive gadget that you must have. Ads are ads—they can often contain overt exaggerations, misrepresentations, and false claims. In an effort to protect consumers and create a culture of awareness, the FDA launched its Bad Ad campaign, which creates a mechanism that allows consumers and health care providers to report ads that are misleading or false. Reports go to the Office of Prescription Drug Promotion. You can report false ads by calling 1-855-RX-BADAD or emailing BadAd@FDA.gov.

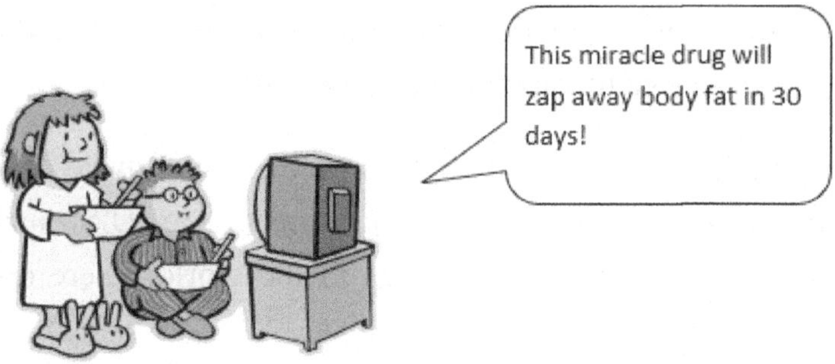

You can also report ads from sales representatives, speaker presentations, TV, or radio, and from written or printed drug information. Although the FDA has limited jurisdiction on ads for over-the-counter products, dietary supplements, and medical devices, you still should be on high alert for false and deceptive advertising.

As you can see, there is a troubling trend in direct-to-consumer prescription drug ads because:

- They are not objective. They often market medicines as if they were a common commodity, like a new car or must-have gadget.
- They push primarily brand-name products that come with a heftier price tag.
- They often use paid actors and celebrities, who lead you to believe that those high-profile people are using those medications and are encouraging you to do the same thing. It is often false and misleading.

Maintaining the integrity of the doctor-patient dynamic is important to the medical profession. We should let doctors do their jobs and diagnose and treat patients without undue influence.

Research and Development Costs

Drug companies spend a lot of money on the research and development of drugs, and, as multinational businesses, they intend to reap positive returns on their investments when those drugs get to market. The cost of research and development of a new drug can top $1 billion; meanwhile, the typical drug company is a for-profit business. In other words, it's a business with shareholders who ultimately want to see profits. Here in America, if a drug is patented, then during the first 7 to 12 years, when the company holds an exclusive patent on the drug, there are no incentives or competition to keep the drug cost down. Drug companies with exclusive patents can set the price tag for their own drugs. Lately, the price tag keeps trending higher. In 2018, the price increases of brand-name drugs more than doubled the price of inflation.[21]

In recent years, the drug manufacturing industry has been accused of "pay-for-delay" tactics, in which brand-name drug companies take generic drug companies to court in efforts to delay release of their generic drugs. Some brands pay the makers of generics to delay the release of their less-expensive generic version of the drug, which would allow the manufacturer to preserve their brand-name market share.

In fact, Americans do tend to use more expensive drugs compared to other developed countries. On average, older Americans use more than four brand-name prescription medications routinely.[22] This is fueled by the increase in new blockbuster drugs and manufacturers discontinuing old generic drugs that happen to cost patients less but provide the company with much lower profit margins. The innovation of new brand-name drugs is valuable, but new blockbuster drugs don't necessarily offer significant advantages or improve outcomes as compared to less expensive generic or therapeutic alternatives. When they do offer significant improvements, the drug prices are set unrealistically high.

To offer a temporary fix for brand-name prescription drug costs, manufacturers introduced rebates that help patients get certain brand-name drugs at a discounted price. These rebate programs come with quite a few limitations that many patients might not qualify for, and, ultimately, they don't change the actual or future price of the drug. They are simply copayment assistance programs that temporarily allow drug manufacturers to pay for some of the cost of the drug. Although patients are happy to take any discounts they can get on their medications, these rebate programs create an illusion of affordability, which, in turn, has continued to push both patients and doctors to use more expensive medicines.

The Growth of Specialized Medicine and the Decline in Primary Care Physicians

Chronic illnesses and the products and services that it takes to care for them make up the majority of health care costs. The key to minimizing those costs is prevention.[23] Every patient's primary care physician (PCP) is essential to patient care, yet PCPs are becoming a dying breed. PCPs perform preventative health services, monitor patients' overall health, and coordinate care with other providers. Unfortunately, The United States currently has a very low number of primary care physicians relative to the size of its population. When compared to 25 other countries, the U.S. ranks 19th in the number of PCPs per population.[24]

At the same time that we are seeing a decline in the number of PCPs, we are seeing tremendous growth in specialized medicine. These days, many doctors are going into specialty fields instead of primary care after they graduate from medical school. As a result, by 2032, it is estimated that there will be a shortage of over 55,000 primary-care physicians in the United States.[25] This is a sobering statistic. Meanwhile, evidence continues to show the impact of chronic health conditions on patients' quality of life and health outcomes. This dynamic creates an unhealthy balance that almost guarantees that patients will receive fragmented and incomplete care. Preventative health care services, such as mammograms, colonoscopies, screenings for blood pressure, diabetes, and cholesterol, immunizations, Pap smears, and general wellness counseling performed by a primary care provider can often detect problems early. And, of course, early detection can mean better long-term outcomes. For patients dealing with chronic health issues, routine follow-up with a primary care physician is essential to managing their health.

Having a PCP involved in patient care is essential to lowering overall costs and ensuring continuity of care for patients. It is an absolute necessity in our ever-so-fragmented health care system.

For-profit Health Care

Most of the institutions involved in our health care system are for-profit, including hospitals, clinics, ambulatory care, health insurance, long-term care facilities, nursing homes, and pharmacies. Most patients access care using their medical health insurance network.

Our health care insurance system is a huge business with significant financial overhead costs. Up to 30% of the costs of health care services go towards the administration of plan benefits.

That means that for every one dollar of health care services you use, 30 cents goes toward administrative costs, which are then passed on to patients through higher premiums and deductibles. For many developed countries, administration costs are closer to 5%. When a fragmented system has plenty of gatekeepers and differing benefits and formularies, as ours does, the cost to operate and maintain it is high. The ultimate bottom line for a "for-profit" business is higher revenue. Ultimately, for-profit businesses are accountable to their shareholders and investors. That means that, until health care companies change their focus from the bottom line to health care outcomes, the cost of health care will continue to increase—and patients and providers will bear most of the burden.

Duplication of Services

In today's health care system, wasteful duplication is rampant. With fewer patients using a primary care physician, patients see multiple doctors who might order duplicate tests and procedures or even duplicate prescriptions. Duplication of medications is an all-too-common issue I see in the pharmacy. Patients should keep records of dates and results of any recent tests, labs, or procedures to make sure those services aren't unnecessarily repeated. If you see a new doctor or specialist, be sure to have your updated medical and prescription records sent over. Always have an up-to-date list of your current medications on hand. Be proactive, be organized, and keep good records to guard against costly replication of services or medications.

Inadequate Continuity of Care

A lot of patients don't have a designated primary care physician, so they seek medical advice from peers, co-workers, family, friends—and the internet. Information from non-medical sources is not always accurate or complete. For many, the community pharmacy becomes their medical home. They can seek medical and drug advice from a pharmacist without the hassle of scheduling an appointment or paying for a consult. Many patients come to me confused, afraid, and helpless, needing advice. Some want me to diagnose and treat their illness or symptoms. I have to remind patients that I am a pharmacist and not a medical doctor. I listen, I observe, I ask questions, and I give my best professional advice. For some, I might recommend an OTC drug if it's appropriate. Others I might encourage to seek the care of a medical doctor.

For the many Americans that don't have insurance, emergency and urgent care services typically become their primary recourse to health care access. As care gets fragmented, it loses efficiency. Patients see different doctors and use multiple pharmacies, and as a result, there's no uniform way for health care providers to centrally access medical records. There is plenty of duplication and redundancy that puts patients at risk.

For care providers, having access to the patient's detailed health and medical history is important to treating patients. Being able to access real-time information about a patient's health history—labs, allergies, procedures, tests, and prescriptions—enables providers to deliver better care. But they typically have to rely on patient self-reporting of medical history, which can be incomplete.

Electronic medical record systems are a useful tool in health care today and are getting more commonplace. For example, a patient recently came into the pharmacy to pick up his medicine. He had been prescribed Atorvastatin 40mg by his cardiologist. As I performed a drug utilization review, the electronic medical record system alerted me that the patient had recently picked up a 20mg prescription for Atorvastatin a few days ago from a different pharmacy. So I called the doctor to verify the prescription and learned that the patient's new dose was 40mg per day. I was able to counsel the patient that he should not take both doses of medications. Since he had just recently picked up the 20 mg dose, I advised him to take two tablets of the 20mg dose per day—equivalent to 40mg per day—and to use up that prescription first. Once he finished that, he could return to the pharmacy to pick up the new prescription.

Electronic prescribing is a step in the right direction, but there is still more that can be done to make systems integrated, centralized, and accessible. Giving pharmacists detailed medical and prescription history is critical to their ability to provide good care now and in the future.

No Regulation of Drug Prices

Unlike some other countries, the United States does not uniformly negotiate or regulate drug prices with drug manufacturers. This means that Americans pay more for their drugs, while other countries that negotiate drug prices often pay less. In the U.S., drug companies get to determine how much their medicines cost, regardless of how high or outrageous the price. A case in point concerns a drug called Daraprim, an antiparasitic drug that used to cost less than $15 per tablet. After the drug was acquired by another drug company, the drug price increased to $750 per tablet![26] The manufacturer of the EpiPen, an epinephrine injection for patients with severe allergies, received backlash from patients and the medical community due to reports of price gouging that resulted in some patients being unable to afford their medicine.

Every day across America, patients wrestle with the inability to afford medications for diabetes, chemotherapy, heart, lung, and neurological conditions. In recent years increases in drug prices have been growing faster than inflation. More and more patients will continue to feel the pinch at the pharmacy counter when paying for their medications.

Higher Cost of Services

In America, we pay for higher-costing services even when there are less expensive alternatives. We often equate high cost with better quality, luxury, and social status. We see celebrities on the cover of magazines or in ads promoting certain products, and we want to use what they use. I find that I have to frequently remind people that care has to be individualized. Sometimes people tell me that they want a medicine because their brother-in-law or aunt or sister uses it. But when it comes to your health, one size simply does not fit all. Your health care decisions should be between you and your health care provider. And at every level of care, choose what is best for *you*—not someone else.

Chapter 9
Anatomy of a Drug Price

By the time that pill lands in your bottle, its cost has gone through a series of negotiations among the manufacturer and private distribution channels, many of which even your pharmacist is unaware. While you pay your pharmacist for the drug, they do not determine how much you pay for it. Let's take a look at some real life scenarios.

~~~~~~~

Pharmacist: The copay on your medicine is $20, ma'am.

Patient: No! No! No! My sister gets the same medication for $10. Why am I paying more?

~~~~~~~

Pharmacist: That'll be $29.99.

Patient: That much for this tiny bottle?! There are only a few tablets inside. Can you at least fill it up with more pills for the same price!

~~~~~~~

Pharmacist: I am sorry to inform you that your insurance does not cover the medication you have been prescribed today.
~~~~~~~

Patient: No! That is not true. My insurance covered the medication just fine when I took it two years ago!

~~~~~~~

Patients often ask why medications cost so much and why costs can vary from pharmacy to pharmacy. The simple answer is that pharmacies don't all pay the same amount for a drug, and the price a pharmacy charges for a drug is based on how much it costs to acquire it. When you pick up your medicine at the pharmacy, the price you are quoted is not an arbitrary number that your pharmacist pulls out of the air. There is a lot that goes into how it is determined. It is a long journey from the drug manufacturer to the pharmacy, and several entities get involved along the way, each one typically marking up the cost.

Let's start at the beginning. The sticker price for a drug, or *manufacturer price*, is determined by the drug manufacturer, the company that makes the drugs. Manufacturers usually use distributers to facilitate the distribution and sale of their drugs. Licensed drug distributors and wholesalers purchase drugs from the manufacturer at a discounted price, the *wholesale price*, often some negotiated percentage off from the listed manufacturer price. Wholesalers often keep a percentage of the discount as profit and pass on the rest of the discount to their clients to build loyalty. They mark up the cost based on their own particular business model or formula. The wholesaler then sells the drugs to other medical entities—such as pharmacies, physician offices, hospitals, and long-term care facilities—which then use their own formulas to determine the retail cost of the drug.

When pharmacies or other medical facilities purchase drugs from the drug wholesaler, their costs can vary. That's because each entity is privately and contractually negotiating its acquisition costs.
~~~~~~~

As a patient, if you don't have insurance, you might have to pay the full retail price for the drug. If you do have insurance, though, the pharmacy bills your insurance company, and you pay your copayment or coinsurance based on your insurance company's negotiated discounted price. When your drugs are covered by insurance, the amount that the pharmacy is reimbursed —as payment for providing the medication to you—is determined by the Pharmacy Benefit Manager (PBM) that your insurance company contracts with to process your prescription benefit. The PBM can bargain with drug manufacturers, on the behalf of your insurance company, for discounts on the cost of the drugs in order to lower the cost of drugs for their insurance members.

The Complex Drug Pathway

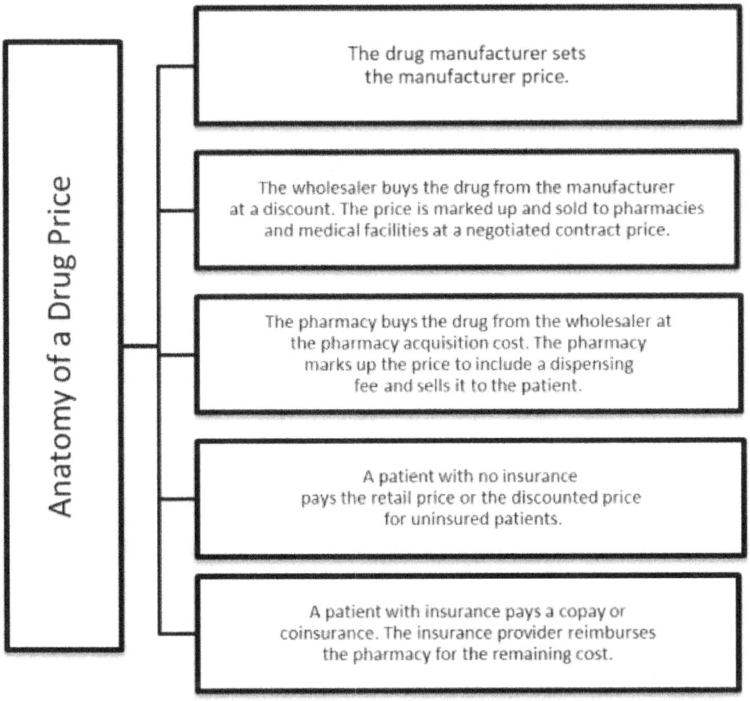

Brands vs. Generic

Whether a drug is classified as a brand or generic can also affect the cost of the drug. The market for brand and generic prescription drugs varies drastically. There is not as much price competition among brand-name drugs because they can only be purchased from one brand manufacturer. Among generic manufacturing companies, however, there is more price competition. Pharmacies with strong buying power are able to purchase directly from generic manufacturers; that can help to drive costs down significantly because the fewer entities involved in distribution, the more savings can be passed down to the patient.

The Drug Price Maze

(This example is for illustrative purposes only. Actual medication costs and pricing contracts will vary.)

- A drug manufacturer determines the list price for Drug X. The list price is based on factors such as the cost of research and development, cost of operations, and the drug's perceived value.

  The list price for 30 tablets of Drug X = $200

- A wholesaler buys the drug from the manufacturer at a price less than the list price due to specific negotiated discounts. For example, if the wholesaler gets a 20% discount, they purchase Drug X for $160. After purchase, the wholesaler might charge a distribution fee to the next buyer.

  $200 – 20% discount + $10 distribution fee = $170

- A pharmacy buys Drug X from the wholesaler at a price based on their negotiated contract. The negotiated price can include discounts and added fees. For example, the pharmacy might acquire the drug for $175

- The pharmacy adds a dispensing fee of $5 to its acquisition costs, so:

  The retail cost becomes $175 + $5 = $180

- A patient that has no insurance pays the retail cost of $180 (or uses available discount programs to lower the cost)

- A patient with insurance pays their copayment or coinsurance payment, such as a copayment of $20 or a coinsurance amount of 20%, or $36.

- Once the patient pays, they can pick up their medicine, and their journey ends.

- However, for the pharmacy, the story isn't quite over. If a patient uses insurance to pay for Drug X, as most Americans do, the pharmacy still needs to be reimbursed by the insurance company's PBM for the cost of providing the drug.

- The pharmacy gets reimbursed based on their negotiated contracts with the insurance company and is at the mercy of the insurance PBM when it comes to the amount they are reimbursed. For example, an insurance PBM might base reimbursement on the listed average wholesale price for Drug X, which might be lower than the pharmacy's retail price

To illustrate the point further, let's say the listed average wholesale price for Drug X is $150. So the pharmacy receives $150 (insurance reimbursement) + $20 (patient copay) for a grand total of $170 as its reimbursement. But the pharmacy retail cost is $180. That means the pharmacy loses $10 in the transaction.

Making matters worse, the PBM subjects the pharmacy to periodic audits and can decide to take back already-issued reimbursements payments on prescriptions that patients have already received, which can cause a pharmacy to be upside-down on dispensed medications. In effect, the pharmacy's cost to provide the drug to the patient can be more than the PBM reimbursement.

This trend is becoming more commonplace and, as a result, many pharmacies operate at a loss. This is the primary reason why so many small independent local pharmacies are going out of business. Small independent pharmacies that were once the cornerstone of American pharmacy services are becoming a dying breed because they lack the unlimited capital and buying power that large blockbuster pharmacy systems have today.

In the drug business, there is little to no transparency about drug costs, resulting in often drastic price differences among pharmacies for similar products.

The fragmentation in the drug supply channel is why many drugs don't have standard and uniform pricing, and why they can cost $5 at one pharmacy and $15 at another. When you shop around for the best price on your prescription drugs, keep in mind that pharmacies with their own distribution channels are often able to bypass the supply chain and buy directly from the manufacturer, which can mean added savings for your medications.

Where the Money Goes

Here in the United States, we spend 20% of the Gross Domestic Profit (GDP) on health care, and most of the money goes towards outpatient and inpatient care, drugs, health insurance, and administration and health investments.[27] Outpatient care includes doctor office visits and same-day medical care, such as emergency department, urgent care, dental care, diagnostic imaging, and clinics. Inpatient care includes hospitals, nursing homes, and long-term care facilities. Health care administration can be costly due to the multiplicity, complexity, and variability of the health insurance market. When services are provided to patients, health care providers are responsible for filing medical claims to get paid for the services provided. With no uniformity in plan administration, providers must first file claims and then wait for reimbursement after care has already been provided. Many health care systems use the services of third-party health care coding and insurance specialists to help navigate the complex terrain of insurance billing and reimbursement. The fee-for-service transaction model of care all but guarantees a complex cost-ridden administration process. Health care administration is so fragmented and complex that even insurance companies contract with benefit management companies, whose job it is to administer the health insurance plan.

Health investment costs include the cost of research, technology, and public health education that are essential to patients and communities. The cost of inpatient care is a significant one for Americans. With the poverty rate at 11% and with millions of people uninsured, when health care issues arise, many people are more likely to end up in the hospital simply because they had limited access to preventative services. The rising cost of drugs, medical devices, and inpatient hospital care accounts for the majority of the increased burden patients have to bear.

There is no doubt that taking care of patients is no simple task. It can be complex and time-intensive. Health care today is comprised of many multidisciplinary providers and care teams, using a variety of systems, diagnostic tools, and technology. Although there are essential costs of patient care, unnecessary costs can be avoided or managed. Finding a balance between care and cost is critical to sustaining a quality health care system that is affordable for everyone. It is something that continues to be a challenge. All providers, too, have a role to play in examining their practices and ensuring the teams and systems they use are in line with the ultimate goal of caring for patients as efficiently as possible.

Chapter 10
The Damaging Effects of Marketing Drugs to Health Care Providers

In order for a drug company to market a prescription drug for a specific condition, clinical studies must show proof of efficacy in treating that condition. It is illegal for them to market drugs for *off-label use*—for conditions other than what the drug is intended and approved to treat. Even so, the practice still takes place. Several whistleblower lawsuits that have been brought against drug manufacturers have shed more light on such practices, and they remind us that the practices do exist in our health system.[28]

The FDA sets parameters for drug companies, including determining which marketing practices it considers illegal. Those practices include:[29]

- marketing drugs in unapproved conditions or symptoms
- marketing drugs in unapproved populations
- marketing drugs in higher doses just to increase sales

At the same time, doctors can use their clinical judgment to decide to prescribe a drug for off-label use if it will benefit the patient. To ensure the efficacy of prescription drugs for the conditions they treat, the FDA monitors drug marketing and takes legal action against companies that break the rules. Federal regulators have recovered billions of dollars in fines from drug manufacturers accused of deceptive off-label marketing.[30] In 2012, GlaxoSmithKline was fined $3 billion for the misbranding of Paxil and Wellbutrin, and Abbot Laboratories was fined $1.5 billion for misbranding Depakote.[31] Avanir Pharmaceuticals, the maker of Nuedexta, was fined over $100 million for paying kickbacks to doctors to boost sales.[32] In 2007, drug manufacturer Purdue was charged with misbranding the drug Oxycontin and paid fines totaling $634 million for misrepresenting the drug's risk of abuse and addiction.[33]

Oxycontin is an opioid medication used to treat pain. It was marketed intensely and was prescribed frequently in the late 90s and early 2000s. Its marketing claimed a low risk of abuse and addiction, which was later proven to be untrue. As a result, the overprescribing of opioid drugs—and oxycontin in particular—has resulted in a serious epidemic of substance abuse and overdosing in numerous communities across the country.

Misbranding is the act of misrepresenting the use or effectiveness of a drug. Health care providers have an ethical obligation to patients to ensure that the drugs that are prescribed are efficacious for the conditions been treated. In an industry where drug companies vie for market share and seek to corner the market, a lot of resources are invested in marketing to prescribers. Drug companies view providers as the gateway to the success of a drug, and drug manufacturers try really hard to sway providers' prescribing habits in their favor. The manufacturers are able to identify and monitor the prescribing habits of providers using data mining practices. Drug manufacturers make it a priority to get on the prescriber's radar and market aggressively in the hopes that when it's time for the doctors to write prescriptions, they choose the marketed one over any other.

Health care providers need to remain aware of the power they hold. With just a few strokes of a pen, they are often making a big decision to start a patient on a drug, and that can have life-altering effects and consequences. It's not just the market share for a drug company that's at stake; it's giving all patients quality care that is safe and free from unethical bias.

It is also common for drug companies to offer prescribers financial incentives when marketing drugs. Data shows that when prescribers receive financial incentives from drug companies, their prescribing habits are affected, and they prescribe more brand-name drugs.[34] The marketing efforts pay off. Data collected from Medicare Part D prescription claims reveal that, for most of the top 50 brand-name drugs, doctors that received financial payments increased their prescribing of the drug compared to doctors who did not.[35]

Providers, therefore, need to be cautious of drug sales representatives that try to influence prescribing habits with gifts, cash incentives, or lavish sponsorships. These are tactics that drug manufacturers have been known to use to sway doctors to prescribe their drugs. Drug sales representatives do whatever they can to sway the provider. They use buzz words and fancy words physicians want to hear. They try to gain trust with their seemingly friendly gestures. They often give freebies like drug samples, stationery, and office supplies, buy lunch, or give expensive gifts and tickets and pay hefty consultation fees. It's all part of the game of building loyalty to the drug brand.

I can often tell when a drug rep has been spending time marketing to a physician. I suddenly see changes in the doctor's prescribing patterns that favor certain brand-name drugs. Then, patients come to the pharmacy with their prescriptions and coupons for the drugs and are often astonished by the cost. I hear things like, "My doctor told me it would only cost $10," but then they are alarmed when the copay is much higher than that. More than likely, the drug rep told the doctor it would cost a certain amount, so that's what the doctor believed to be true. But the drug rep or doctor does not typically know the type of pharmacy insurance plan or the plan benefit the patient actually has. When the patient arrives at the pharmacy, then, the pharmacist looks like the bad guy when they are the bearer of bad news. They have to explain to the patient why the copay isn't what the doctor said it would be after all.

Doctors might mean well by handing their patients manufacturer coupons, and I applaud their genuine attempt to try to save patients some money. But a brand-name manufacturer copayment card might not change a patient's deductible or coinsurance amount and still leaves the patient paying a hefty drug price. Instead of unintentionally quoting the patient the wrong medication price, a provider that is giving a patient a drug coupon with their prescription should inform the patient that it *might* help lower the cost of the medicine and that they should check with their pharmacist for specific copay pricing to find out for sure.

As a pharmacist, it is often frustrating for me to see the cost burden that patients and health systems bear because of naïve practices. I encourage physicians to use local community pharmacists as a resource for drug information and cost instead of drug sales reps that are so far removed from the frontlines of care. A drug rep is the sales force for a drug company and will often be biased towards that specific brand or product. The pharmacist is a more qualified and objective resource when it comes to drug information and pricing.

Drug reps come prepared when they talk to providers. They have prescribing data from drug companies that purchased it from pharmacies or third-party data collectors. The data tells them which drugs doctors are prescribing and in what areas. Drug companies then use the information to understand a doctor's prescribing habits, and they're very good at it—regardless of the efficacy or cost-effectiveness of the products they sell.

Pharmacists get visits from drug reps, too. I don't mind the occasional visits that provide me with informative drug literature. I welcome materials that provide the drug parameters that are important for me to know when I consult with doctors or counseling patients. But I do find troubling the aggressive sales tactics that some drug reps use. In one encounter, a drug rep tried to convince me to order a stockpile of a new brand-name drug. I asked him why I would want to order a stockpile of product that I have never dispensed before when I could simply order it as needed.

"Well," he said, "just in case."

I had to pass!

The Importance of Making Informed Choices

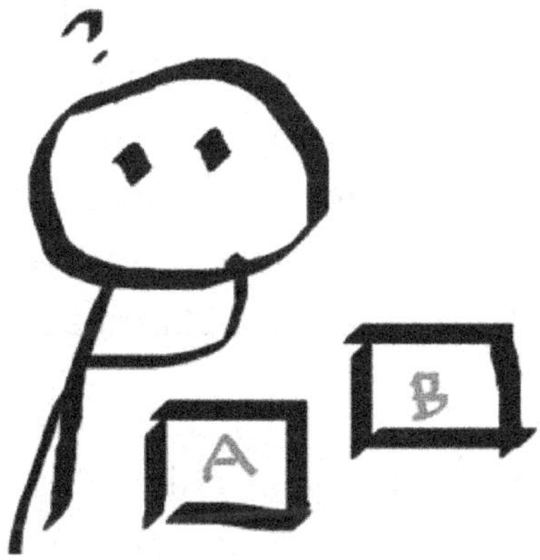

As health care costs continue to increase, more and more of the cost of care will be passed on to patients. It is projected that health care spending will make up 25% of the GDP in the next few years. It is critical for patients to make informed choices when faced with health care decisions.

As a patient, you are faced with important decisions related to your health care. Sometimes, you will have to do so during emotional times, such as the birth of a child, a critically-ill relative in the hospital, surgery, a cancer treatment, or a new medicine to be prescribed. As difficult as it may be, you should try to approach decisions with an objective mind. Doing so will save you time and money. When making health care decisions for you or for others, it will be very helpful if you:

- know the facts
- know your options
- do your research and read the literature provided
- ask questions
- get a second opinion, if necessary
- make an informed decision

Do not be afraid or intimidated—that white coat can do that to patients! Health care providers, pharmacists included, tend to use a lot of medical jargon that many patients find intimidating and confusing. It is not intentional; it is part of providers' medical training and a hard habit to break—especially when talking to patients. If you are unsure, ask for clarification. Speak up and be heard.

One thing you can do prior to your visit with a health care provider is to think about the questions or concerns you have prior to your visit and write them down. If you don't understand the information you've been given, say so. It is OK. Your pharmacist is your health care advocate. If you need more information about a medicine or simply want drug literature prior to taking a medication, just ask.

Many of us have had to make important health care decisions at one point or another. We want to know which doctor, hospital, pharmacy, or procedure we should use. Most of us try to make the right choices. For example, one of the decisions I had to make as a patient was whether or not to do a natural birth for my youngest children. My first child was born by Caesarean section (C-section), and my doctor recommended doing the same thing for the birth of my three youngest children. But I disagreed because I had no preexisting health issues or complications, and my pregnancies were not high-risk. I chose a natural birth, knowing the cost and recovery time would be significantly less than it would be with a Caesarean section. Born years apart, all of my youngest children were born naturally —with no complications.

I actually made the tough decision to change doctors mid-pregnancy due to the pressure I was feeling from my doctor. I respected my doctor immensely, however, I chose to change doctors and get a second opinion because I felt it was not the best decision for my circumstances.

Much later, my doctor and I discussed the challenges facing our professions as health care providers. She is an OB/GYN doctor; I am a pharmacist. My doctor told me frankly that she had to change how she practices due to a case in the past that caused her serious anxiety and fear of liability. Interestingly enough, a C-section is often viewed as simple and routine, while natural births can be seen as complicated and unpredictable. C-sections account for a third of all childbirths, and among women who have had a previous C-section, the rate is 90%.

I have to admit that, with all of my pregnancies, the pressure from providers to choose a C-section was extremely high. I was always very conscious and puzzled by this. That is not to say that mothers who elect for a C-section are wrong. Child-birth is a uniquely personal experience for every mother. But the reality is that mothers are increasingly electing C-sections—even for uncomplicated births—partly because it is part of the unquestioned narrative they get from their providers and hospitals.[36]

This practice of defensive medicine is highly ingrained in our health care system. With the infusion of technology and modern medicine, the practice of defensive care sometimes leads to a greater propensity to perform more surgical intervention. Yes, surgical intervention is needed when warranted, and there is no doubt that technology provides us with new tools in diagnosis and treatment. However, patients always deserve an unbiased narrative of what their options are. Giving them this empowers them and provides the tools to navigate their care as well as possible. It is always important for patients to make informed choices on health care decisions that affect them.

The reality of our health care system is that a simple procedure or health issue can leave people with a huge financial burden. I began writing this book soon after my 10-year-old was born. We finally finished paying off all the medical bills from his delivery about the time he was starting to walk. Even though I had medical insurance, our out-of-pocket medical expenses were significant, and, like many Americans, we had to put our medical bills on a monthly payment plan.

Fortunately for me, I have health insurance. But 15% of Americans—close to 48 million people—do not have health insurance. If you are fortunate enough to have insurance, imagine not having it. Seeing the itemized bill from a hospital, doctor, or pharmacy can leave a person in a state of shock and disbelief. Many uninsured patients just delay care due to their concerns about the costs. Some even ration care or medicines because of cost. Unfortunately, rationing medication is not a good solution. Rationing your medicines can be dangerous, especially for patients with chronic conditions such as diabetes, high blood pressure, and lung disease.[37]

If you are concerned about how much you spend on health care and medicines, you are not alone. Many Americans are drowning in medical debt. It has become a significant factor in personal bankruptcy in the U.S.; reports show between 46 to 62% of personal bankruptcy filings in the U.S. are due to medical debt.

We wonder why our health care costs are growing at such an alarming rate. It is partly because of the health care choices we make, and in some cases, the choices that are beyond our control and are often made for us. Why is it that Americans spend more on health care than any other developed country, but among the same group, our health outcomes are among the lowest? Part of the reason is that some of the health services we spend our money on are not improving our health outcomes and might be unsafe.

Quick Rx Tip: One of the most important things you can do as a patient is to be an informed consumer. You should remain engaged in your health care by doing your research, knowing the facts, understanding your options, asking questions, and making informed choices.

Knowledge Checkpoint

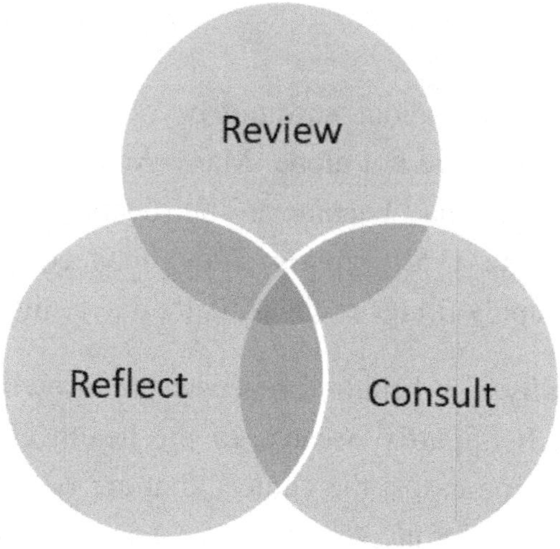

REVIEW: From the preceding chapters, you now know the ways that prescriptions can be transmitted to the pharmacy and the review process they go through prior to dispensing. You reviewed tips to help you better understand the instructions on your pill bottle and gained a better understanding of the reasons why medications and health care costs are on the rise. You then took a closer look behind the variability in drug prices and the factors that determine the price of a drug. You gained a better understanding of the marketing pressures that doctor's face and the importance of working collaboratively with your provider to make informed choices on matters pertaining to your care.

REFLECT: Take a moment to reflect on what you have learned and then answer these questions: Do you have any concerns about your medication instructions? Are you shocked by the cost of your medicines? How will you use the added insight to improve your health literacy? Think about a health-related concern or decision you are currently facing. Do you understand the facts? Do you know your options? Have you done your research? Do you need a second opinion? How can you use the added insight to make an informed decision?

CONSULT: Now, write down all your questions or concerns. Then, take the next opportunity to discuss them with your health care provider.

Chapter 11
Everything You Need to Know to Save Time and Money at the Pharmacy

Going to the pharmacy can be a very routine experience, but it can also be extremely confusing. Who wants to waste their time and money at the pharmacy counter? No one! Here are the things you really should acquaint yourself with before you head to the pharmacy counter. They are the "nut and bolts" of what you need to know to save time and money.

Q & A. Your Questions Answered!

• ***When my doctor writes a prescription, isn't my insurance required to pay for it?***

No, when you are issued a prescription, this does not guarantee that your insurance company will cover it. Your insurance company is not obligated to cover a medication written by your doctor. However, don't worry; there are always other options to remedy this situation.

• ***What are the best insurance plans?***

Patients often want to know which ones are the best insurance plans. The answer is that there isn't a best insurance plan or company, so to speak. The right one for you is based on your specific situation and needs as a patient. During your health insurance enrollment period, you have to decide which plan is best suited for you based on your circumstances and preferences.

To find the one best for you, prior to your insurance open enrollment period, make a list of what you value most in a health insurance plan and use it as a guide to select a plan that best meets your criteria. You should take into consideration the types of services each plan offers, the deductibles, copayments, and coinsurance. If you have been using a specific doctor or pharmacy and want to continue doing so, look closely to ensure these providers are in the preferred network before deciding which insurance plan to use. Also, pay close attention to the services that are not covered and decide whether or not that is a deal-breaker for you. You can also look up the insurance company consumer rating online to assist in your decision-making. However, not all consumers have a say in deciding which insurance plan to choose since, for many, that decision is made by an employer.

• ***What is a prescription refill, and if I need it, how do I request one?***

A prescription refill means that the doctor has authorized you to reorder your medicine when it's needed. If you have refills available on your prescription, you can request a refill in person, by phone, or through available digital platforms. Simply check your prescription bottle to see if there are any authorized refills listed on your bottle. If you are unsure, simply contact the pharmacy to check if you have refills on file.

When you do not have any refills left for your medicine, your pharmacy can contact your doctor on your behalf, or you can contact your provider directly. Many providers have a dedicated medication refill line or online portal for patients to notify the doctor that a refill is needed. Refill request policies can vary, so be sure to ask your doctor how refill requests are handled. It can take 24 to 72 hours or even longer for a response from the prescribing doctor. If your refill has not been approved after that time, it is best to call your doctor for advice.

• ***Why did the hospital or emergency room doctor deny my refill request?***

In-patient hospital and emergency room doctors do not usually authorize refills after you have finished the supply of medicines and original refills you were issued. If you have been discharged from a hospital with medicine, you will be instructed to follow up with your primary care provider or a specialist before you run out so that there is continuity of your health care and medications.

• ***Why do my pills look different?***

If your medicine's bottle or packaging looks very different from the last time you picked it up, don't be alarmed. The same medication might have a different appearance than your last refill because there has been a change in the drug manufacturer of your medicine. With generic medications, different drug manufacturers can produce the same generic equivalent drug. These drugs are bio-identical but might not have the same physical appearance, such as color, size, and shape. And, although the same generic drugs might have different manufacturers, they are required to have equivalent potency, bioavailability, and safety. For patients on routine medications, the pharmacist tries their best to use a specific manufacturer on each refill, but drug industry supply-and-demand issues make it logistically impossible for that to occur all the time. The pharmacist will make an effort to notify you of a manufacturer change, but due to the volume of prescriptions being processed, it, too, can be logistically impossible. If you're concerned, don't hesitate to call your pharmacist and ask why your pills look different.

• ***What can I do if I don't like the taste of my medication?***

If you don't like the taste of your medicine, there's something you can do about it. Some pharmacies have flavoring services for liquid medicines, which can be especially helpful for young children. Check with your pharmacist if your liquid medicine can be flavored. There are also over-the-counter flavoring sprays that can be used to coat the mouth prior to taking pills to make swallowing more palatable.

• ***I need a quick and easy drug test. What can I do?***

You can purchase over-the-counter drug tests from the pharmacy for discreet at-home use. They can test for substances like ecstasy, methamphetamines, opioids, cocaine, heroin, and other substances.

• ***Why are drug names so hard to pronounce?***

Deciphering drug names can be a tough one. Even pharmacy professionals stumble every now and then. Many drug names, especially generic drugs, are derived from and often referred to by their chemical ingredient name. The process of creating a drug name is a blend of art and science. But don't be intimidated by the bizarre drug name of your medication. If you have trouble remembering how to say the names of your medication, you are not alone. Most patients experience the same frustration. Simply ask for help, and the pharmacist will educate you on the proper pronunciation.

• ***What are vaccines? Do Pharmacists give vaccines?***

A vaccine is a type of medicine that protects you from a specific illness by stimulating the immune system. Receiving a vaccine is also referred to as an "immunization." A vaccine can contain a tiny deactivated or weakened component of a virus or bacteria that causes your body to produce antibodies. Antibodies are cells that help the body recognize and fight infections so that, upon exposure to disease, sickness is avoided or significantly minimized. Vaccines are typically used to prevent disease. The most common vaccine administered by the pharmacist is the annual flu shot or influenza vaccine. Pharmacists in many states also have vaccine administration programs, where pharmacists, under a supervising doctor protocol or with a doctor's prescription, administer vaccines that protect against diseases such as pneumonia, shingles, coronavirus, tetanus, diphtheria, pertussis, varicella, measles, mumps, rubella, hepatitis, and many others.

• ***What are the pros and cons of using a prescription mail order service?***

If your insurance company allows you to use a mail-order service for your refill, here's what you should know. Mail-order prescriptions let you get your prescription delivered through the mail using a mail-order pharmacy, which can offer 90-day prescription incentives on maintenance drugs—often lower than what you'd pay at a retail pharmacy. To take advantage of the program, call your insurance company or use their website to register for the service. The mail-order pharmacy you use will need to obtain a new prescription from your doctor, or you might be able to transfer your existing prescription from your retail pharmacy. When using a mail-order pharmacy, you should expect one to two weeks of processing time. Remember: never wait until you are completely out of pills to request a mail-order prescription since shipping delays can occur.

• ***The mail-order prescription I requested hasn't arrived and I am out of pills! What should I do?***

This is a very common situation. Have your doctor send over an emergency prescription to your local pharmacy to get you by until you receive your prescription mail order delivery. A two-week emergency prescription is typically sufficient. Then, notify the pharmacist, too. The pharmacist might need to request an emergency approval from your insurance company.

• ***I have a medicine that is not covered by my insurance. My doctor says I need it but I cannot afford it. What can I do?***

Have your doctor seek prior authorization approval. This is a process by which your doctor directly petitions the insurance company to cover a medication for you. It is necessary when the doctor prescribes a medication that is being denied by the insurance company and involves completing necessary forms and providing supporting medical documentation to the insurance.

• ***What is step therapy or prerequisite therapy, and why is it needed for me to receive my medication?***

Step therapy or prerequisite therapy refers to criteria that your insurance company might have, requiring you to use a less costly drug or a preferred medication first before they cover one that is more expensive or not preferred.

• ***What is a quantity limit, and why am I not getting the complete amount of medicine that my doctor prescribed?***

A quantity limit happens when your insurance company limits how much medicine is *dispensed*, which is different than the quantity prescribed by the doctor. For some drugs, such as those used to treat erectile dysfunction, migraine, insomnia, pain, and other conditions, your insurance company formulary might restrict you to a specific quantity of medication that is covered every month. Any amount above that quantity will result in a denied claim. Here are some examples:

Your doctor wrote a prescription for 30 tablets of Sildenafil for erectile dysfunction, your insurance company might only cover eight tablets per month.

Your doctor wrote a prescription for 30 tablets of Rizatriptan for migraines, your insurance company might only cover 12 tablets per month.

Your doctor wrote a prescription for a three-month supply—90 capsules—of Fluoxetine for depression, your insurance company might only over 30 capsules per month, limiting you to a one-month supply each time.

If your medication has a quantity limit, and you decide you must have the entire quantity prescribed by the doctor, your doctor may have to seek a prior authorization for that quantity or you can pay for it out-of-pocket.

• ***What if I need a medication after hours?***

Some pharmacies have locations that offer extended, late, or 24-hour pharmacy services at select locations. If you get discharged from the hospital after hours, you might want to consider filling your prescription at the facilities' outpatient pharmacy, if available. Hospitals have their own in-house pharmacy, so it might be a good idea to get the hospital pharmacy to process your prescriptions. That way, you have all your needed medications before you leave the facility.

• ***Why do I need a photo identification to get over the counter medications?***

In certain cases, you may need to show identification to get a cold medicine. In many states, common cold, sinus, and cough medications that contain pseudoephedrine are kept behind the pharmacy counter. Products containing pseudoephedrine can be abused illicitly and are used to make methamphetamines, a street drug. Because of this, sales of these products are regulated. Some states have even classified them as controlled substances. Pharmacies are also required to keep a record of all pseudoephedrine sales. That's why you must show identification and sign for such purchases.

• ***I lost my medicine, what do I do?***

It happens! You've searched high and low and cannot find it. You might have left it in the hotel room, in the rental car, or forgotten it in a box somewhere while you were moving. You might have spilled it in the sink while you were trying to take your medicine. Or maybe it fell in the toilet. We've heard it all!

Any time you lose your medication, call your pharmacy and notify them of the circumstances. Some insurance plans might allow for an exception to be made for lost prescriptions, and your pharmacy can contact them for a lost prescription approval. If you don't have a refill on file, then a refill request can be sent to your doctor. If your insurance company does not cover lost prescriptions, you will have to decide whether to pay for them out-of-pocket or not.

• ***My medicine was stolen, what should I do?***

It is a good idea to file a police report, especially if a narcotic or controlled medicine is involved. Then call the pharmacy and notify them of your circumstances. If you have refills, your pharmacy can try to contact your doctor and insurance company for an early refill approval on a stolen medicine. If your insurance company does not cover the cost of replacing stolen prescriptions, then you will have to pay out-of-pocket for your medicine. Limitations do apply for controlled medications. You might also have to provide documentation to validate a stolen prescription claim.

• ***I simply want to know how much a medicine will cost with my insurance. Do I need a prescription?***

Yes, your pharmacy does not process a prescription through your insurance company without a valid prescription on record, even if you simply just want a price check. Doing so may be considered fraud. The pharmacist can provide you with the retail cost of the medicine. If you want a price check with the insurance and do not have a prescription yet, then the best thing to do is to contact your prescription insurance company directly for a price quote or have your doctor write you a prescription.

• ***I have a prescription at another pharmacy, but I want to know how much this medicine costs with you using my insurance?***

Without a prescription on file, the pharmacist cannot legally bill your insurance plan, even for a price check. The pharmacist would have to first transfer the prescription from the other pharmacy. Once the prescription transfer is complete, then it can be processed and the price provided to you with no obligation to purchase.

• ***Can I get my pets prescriptions at the pharmacy, too?***

Yes, your pharmacist can dispense medications for your pets, too. Some prescriptions from veterinarians can be filled by a pharmacist and cost you a whole lot less than getting them filled at the vet's office. Simply ask the veterinarian to issue you a paper prescription that you can give to your pharmacist.

What's Taking So Long?

To protect patients from harm, pharmacists must verify and review every single detail about a prescription. There are many, many times that a pharmacist comes across an issue and has to call the prescriber to discuss and remedy it. Patient wait times might be extended during those times as the pharmacist might not be able to complete another incoming or pending order in the meantime. Trust that the pharmacist gives the same care, consideration, and caution to every patient equally—and that is why it might take some extra time to finish an order.

Don't be alarmed if a prescription has not been received or is not ready when you expected. The pharmacist retrieves prescriptions periodically throughout the day, and they are processed in the order that they arrive. Electronic prescriptions (E-Rx) are commonly used by doctors to send orders. Your doctor might tell you that your order will be sent electronically, but electronic orders can have processing delays due to software system issues and high volume, resulting in a delay in getting to your pharmacy. If the pharmacy did not receive your electronic order, notify the doctor's office as soon as possible.

While there are thousands of prescription drugs available on the market, not every one of them is on the pharmacy's shelves, either. The medicine your doctor ordered for you might not be available on the same day. If not, your pharmacist can place an order for your medicine, and that might take a few days to arrive. Some medications commonly have supply issues, too, and that can delay the arrival of your medication.

Every patient deserves to be treated with dignity and respect, even those who might need extra time at the pharmacy counter. Show kindness even when the patient ahead of you is taking extra time. Pharmacists try to give the same care, attention, and consideration to everyone. At the same time, there is no room for error with medicines. Please be patient.

Every single bottle or package that you receive must be manually reviewed by the pharmacist for safety, completeness, accuracy, dose appropriateness, and other drug or allergy interactions. They have to do that each time they fill a prescription. In other words, delays will occur if your pharmacist detects any adverse drug interactions, allergies, or contraindications or if the prescription is incomplete or inaccurate.

For example, if you have a penicillin allergy on file and your pharmacist receives an order of penicillin for you, they will not fill it. The pharmacist will reach out to your doctor to notify them of this important allergy history and request a change in your medicine, to one that is a safer alternative for you.

Or perhaps, if you have a codeine allergy on file and your doctor prescribed acetaminophen with codeine, your pharmacist will place the prescription on hold and want to speak with your doctor to notify them of your allergy history, so you end up with a safe alternative. In addition, there might be an insurance approval issue that has to be resolved in the event that the insurance denies your medication coverage. The pharmacist has no control over most of these delays but will work diligently to resolve them for you.

It is not always possible for the pharmacists to predict or anticipate the types of hiccups you may experience at the pharmacy as they accept and receive orders as they are sent or turned in. They must navigate each medication order with caution and concern because every patient's health is the number one priority. Patience helps everyone.

For Traveling

According to data from the United States State Department, about 2,500 Americans get arrested each year at the airport while traveling outside the country, and 30% of these arrests are medication-related.[38] A few years ago, I had a patient whose vacation turned into a nightmare after been arrested at an airport outside the United States. It took legal maneuvering from lawyers and help from the U.S. State Department before a release was secured.

When you travel out of the country with medications, make sure you have the necessary documentation, especially if your medications are narcotic or controlled substances. Be thorough in your recordkeeping. You can have your doctor write a letter for you describing your health conditions and the medications you are taking. Carry this letter with you for the entire duration of your travel.

Bring a copy of your prescriptions; you can obtain them from your pharmacist. Also, keep your medications in their original bottles along with the drug information that came with them.

Bring just enough medication for your stay; do not take more than a 30-day supply. Traveling with excessive amounts of controlled medicines on international travel—even with a valid prescription—might place you in violation of international or country-specific laws and can have serious consequences such as detention or arrest outside the United States.

If you are traveling outside the U.S. and you take medicines that are considered narcotic or controlled substances, be sure to do your research to ensure you are compliant with all applicable laws pertaining to all the countries you will be stopping in. You can also call the embassy of the country prior to your departure and inquire about specific protocols related to traveling with prescription medications. Most embassies have websites where you can find all of the information you need.

If you are planning to travel out of town, it's best to notify your pharmacy that you need accommodations for an early refill. Some insurance plans allow for an exception to be made for travel or vacation, especially if you are traveling out of the country.

Don't wait until the last minute when you're on your way to the airport to request a travel supply! Start the process at least a week or two ahead of time. Here's why:

Your pharmacy might need to get refill approval from your doctor, then contact your insurance company to request a travel authorization on your medication. They might also need to order more of the medicine to cover your travel supply. If your insurance company doesn't pay for travel supplies, you might have to pay out-of-pocket for your medicine or wait to fill your medication when you arrive at your destination—if you're traveling within the United States.

When traveling within the U.S, many community pharmacies have locations in other cities and states, and their medication record system is electronically stored and shared among them. That means that if you use the same pharmacy chain, you might be able to fill your prescription anywhere in the United States.

When traveling within the U.S, if your pharmacy does not have a location where you're going, then you can request a manual transfer to another pharmacy of your choice, in which case, the prescription records will be transferred manually via telephone or fax. Remember that when transferring prescriptions, state and federal laws apply that can limit or prevent the process.

Keeping Costs Down

If your insurance company doesn't cover a medication you need, find out how much it costs. The idea is to be reasonable, objective and explore your options. If the medication is relatively inexpensive and within your budget, it might be wise to go ahead and pay for it out-of-pocket and keep your sanity. Do you really want to battle the insurance company over a medication that costs $15 out-of-pocket and is not covered by your insurance? However, if the cost of your drug is too expensive and way out of your budget, then having the doctor change it to something less expensive or pursuing a prior authorization with the insurance company might be better options.

As much as it is hard to comprehend, a large portion of our health care system is made up of for-profit private businesses, including pharmacies. Whether it is a pharmacy, insurance company, doctor, drug manufacturer, health clinic, or hospital, many are in the business of getting people healthy and making money too. Whether or not this is an ideal model for health care is certainly debatable, but this is the reality of our health care system, and the more we recognize it, the better we can deal with it.

Some pharmacies market discounted, low-cost generics or free medications using their own in-house drug-specific pharmacy and don't use your insurance company. But not all pharmacies have these programs. If you paid $4 at one pharmacy, it doesn't mean you can pay just $4 anywhere else.

Why does your medicine cost so much even when you're only getting a few pills? Drug manufacturers spend millions of dollars on research and development of drugs, and part of that cost is passed on to the consumer. Patients who do not have insurance might have to pay a higher cost for drugs. For those that have insurance, the insurance company determines your cost-sharing amount based on your specific plan benefit.

Check with your pharmacist to see if your pharmacy offers prescription discount programs that you might qualify for to help save money on your medications.

Handling Refills

Know which medicines you need and what you are picking up at the pharmacy before you check out. You can politely ask, "What medicine am I getting today?" Or "May I review what I am getting today?" Many patients use automatic refill services, which means that some medicines can refill automatically even if you don't need them. At checkout, ask to confirm which medicines you are picking up before you leave the pharmacy.

If you are sending a friend or family member to pick up your medicines, make sure they know what they are getting and for whom.

It's best to verify that your medicine is ready by calling ahead or using available digital services before you head over to the pharmacy. Insurance and drug manufacturer supply issues commonly delay orders.

Try to plan ahead. Do not wait until the last minute to request a refill, especially when you are in a hurry. There can be unanticipated hiccups when you wait to request a refill at the last minute. You might not have any refills remaining, or the medicine might not be available at the time, which can cause added stress to overcome.

When your doctor denies your medication refill request, remember that your pharmacist does not have the power to override this denial. Asking the pharmacist to go against your doctor's orders is futile. If your doctor denies your medication refill, you should contact your doctor immediately for further instruction. Before you run out of medication, be sure to follow up with your primary care doctor to ensure continuity of any medicines you need.

After you order a refill, pick up your medicine within a reasonable amount of time. A pharmacy will typically hold your ordered medications for you for one to two weeks. The pharmacy cannot keep your medicines ready indefinitely. Do not expect a medicine you ordered over a month ago to be ready to go when you arrive. If you do not pick up your medicine within the pharmacy's stand-by period, it will be returned. The pharmacy does this to comply with insurance billing requirements. Not to worry, you can always reorder your medicines again when you need them.

When you call the pharmacist and ask that "all" of your prescriptions be refilled, expect the pharmacist to ask you to clarify which medications you need. The pharmacist needs to know the names and usually the prescription number for each one you need in order to ensure you get the right medications. Every medication that your doctors have prescribed for you in the past year or two is on your medication chart. Prepare for the call, and have the exact names or prescription numbers from your bottles before you dial. This is for your safety. Sadly, thousands of patients die each year from preventable medication errors that occur at the ordering stage.[39] Do not be a statistic.

If your doctor told you to increase the dosage of your medication, you might need to refill it sooner. For example, if you were taking one capsule two times a day of Gabapentin 300mg, but your doctor just told you to increase it to three times a day, you need to alert your pharmacy. The pharmacist might need to call your insurance company if your prescription claim is denied.

When the doctor increases your dose soon after you picked up a recent supply of the same medication, the insurance plan might not pay for another order right away. If that happens, continue to take your medication—at the new dose your doctor instructed you to take—and return to the pharmacy a few days before your supply runs out to get your new prescription.

Sometimes, your insurance company will give your pharmacy the next available refill date on a medicine, which your pharmacy can provide to you. Make a note of the date on your calendar and return to request a refill then.

Whenever your doctor changes the way you take your medication, be sure to ask your doctor to write you a new prescription with the new instructions. The pharmacist must have the new prescription on record to make any changes to your medication record and also to call your insurance company for approval, if necessary.

Helping The Elderly

For best results and fewer problems, elderly patients should have a designated caretaker or health care proxy to assist with their health care.

A health care proxy is someone who is legally authorized to make health care decisions for a patient. This is especially important when there is a transition of care, such as during discharge from the hospital or entry into a nursing home. At these times, medication changes often occur, and they should be monitored carefully. There will be medicines to stop, new ones to begin, and dosages might change.

The pharmacist offers counseling on these changes, but an elderly patient might forget them, which is why a caretaker should be available to assist with medication compliance.

When an elderly patient's medications change, someone might need to go through their supply cabinet and discard old medicines so that the patient doesn't accidentally take discontinued or duplicate ones. This principle also applies to patients with disabilities or special circumstances. In fact, all of us should go through our medicine stash periodically and discard those that are expired or have been discontinued!

Pharmacy Etiquette

The pharmacy's drive-through window is for prescription and medication-related transactions. It is proper etiquette to come inside and do your personal shopping, or use other options like curb-side pick up or instant delivery. This helps ensure reasonable wait times for all patients.

The pharmacist consultation counter is for medication-related needs. In other words, your pharmacist might be too polite to tell you, but checking out a basket-full of groceries at the pharmacist counter when there are sick patients waiting to get their medications is not considered appropriate. When checking out purchases that are not medicine-related, try to use other checkout counters located in the store. Holding up the pharmacist for non-medication-related issues can be hard on those in need.

Drug Shortages Happen

Medications are sometimes in short supply for days, weeks, and sometimes even months, which would mean that your pharmacist might not be able to dispense your medication to you. One thing you can do is try to transfer your prescription to another pharmacy that has it available. But if the backorder problem is nationwide, it might affect all pharmacies in your area, and your medication won't be available anywhere. If that occurs, your doctor might have to change your prescription to an alternative drug that's available.

Nationwide, many pharmacies and hospitals have to deal with managing drug shortages of important medications—it's a huge headache for doctors, nurses, pharmacists, and patients. The Food and Drug Administration tracks national drug shortages every year. At one point or another, hundreds of drugs have had significant supply problems that have affected the supply chain, including:[40]

Atenolol	High blood pressure
Dorzolamide eye solution	Glaucoma
Dorzolamide/Timolol eye solution	Glaucoma
Ofloxacin ear and eye solution	Infection
Sumatriptan tablets and injection	Migraine
Carbidopa/Levodopa ER tablets	Parkinson's disease
Ciprofloxacin eye solution and oral suspension	Infection
Oseltamivir capsules and suspension	Influenza infection
Furosemide tablet and injection	Diuretic, hypertension
Heparin injection	Blood clots
Indomethacin capsules	Pain/inflammation
Mupirocin cream and nasal ointment	Topical infection
Amino acids	Nutrition
IV fluids (dextrose, sodium chloride)	Fluids to deliver intravenous medications
Epinephrine injection	Anaphylactic reaction
Folic Acid injection	Vitamin
Guanfacine tablets	High blood pressure, attention deficit hyperactivity disorder
Scopolamine transdermal patch	Motion sickness
Theophylline ER tablets and capsules	Asthma
Benzonatate capsules	Cough
Leflunomide tablets	Rheumatoid arthritis
Lorazepam injection	Anxiety, agitation
Meperidine injection	Pain
Methadone injection	Pain
Morphine injection	Pain
Pantoprazole injection	Acid reflux
Promethazine injection	Nausea/vomiting
Tamsulosin	Enlarged prostate
Vancomycin injection	Infection

Recombinant Zoster Vaccine	Shingles vaccine
Promethazine with Dextromethorphan syrup	Cough and cold
Olmesartan	High blood pressure
Olmesartan/hydrochlorothiazide	High blood pressure
Losartan/hydrochlorothiazide	High blood pressure
Valsartan/hydrochlorothiazide	High blood pressure
Buspirone	Anxiety
Dicyclomine	Irritable bowel syndrome
Hydroxyzine Pamoate	Antihistamine
Methocarbamol	Muscle spasms
Methyldopa	High blood pressure
Nystatin suspension	Fungal infection
Valsartan	High blood pressure
Haloperidol	Antipsychotic
Prednisone eye suspension	A steroid used to treat eye irritation and inflammation
Temazepam	Insomnia
Levetiracetam	Seizures
Amphetamine and Dextroamphetamine	Attention deficit hyperactivity disorder
Azithromycin	Infection
Diltiazem	High blood pressure
Famotidine	Heartburn

More Ways to Save Time

- Know your pharmacy's operating hours.
- The pharmacy is your medical home. Get to know your pharmacist and build a patient-pharmacist relationship. You should have a designated pharmacy to handle your medication needs. Unless you have an emergency or extenuating circumstance, drugstore hopping is not safe. Your pharmacist needs to have access to your complete prescription history to provide you with the best medical care.
- Be prepared to ask questions and make informed choices—not emotional ones.
- The pharmacist is your advocate and always has your best interest in mind. Give them the facts, ask for their help, and they will do the best they can to help you.
- Always identify yourself to the pharmacist by giving your name and date of birth. The pharmacy might ask you to verify other personal information before speaking about sensitive information.
- Do not assume that the pharmacist knows you simply by the sound of your voice. A pharmacist can dispense hundreds of prescriptions a day, and it is common for patients to have similar-sounding names and birth dates. You will be routinely asked to verify your identity or the identity of the patient in question. This is the protocol, and it is for your safety.
- If your family uses the same pharmacy as you, add important identifiers to patient accounts such as middle initials, middle names, junior, senior, or twin when

applicable to help differentiate family members that share similar names and to help prevent medication errors.

- When requesting medical records, have a photo identification readily available. If you are requesting medical records for another adult, you might be asked to provide a power of attorney to comply with privacy laws.
- If your prescription insurance company uses a *select preferred pharmacy network*, your prescriptions will only be covered if you receive them from a preferred pharmacy provider. If you have one of these preferred network plans, make sure the pharmacy you turned in your prescription to is in the network. When you drop off at a non-preferred pharmacy provider, the prescription might not be covered; otherwise, all of your running around and waiting in line would be for nothing. Many times, patients who aren't aware of their select preferred pharmacy requirement can't afford to pay out-of-pocket for their medications and have to then transfer it out or take back their hardcopy prescription and start the process all over again at a different pharmacy. It is not a fun experience! It can be a huge waste of time and resources.

Get Technology to Work for You

Use technology to your advantage. When you get your insurance card, use your phone and take a picture of the front and back of your insurance card. That way, if you lose your physical card, you have an electronic image saved. This quick tip is very helpful if you have multiple dependents and only received one or two insurance cards.

Find other ways to use technology to save you time and money at the pharmacy. Many digital platforms that give you access to your medication history, allow you to order refills, check on the status of your prescriptions, look up drug prices, and register for drug discount cards or copayment assistance cards with just a click of a button.

Here's a great example. Recently, a patient turned in a prescription for an expensive specialty drug that would have cost him a couple of hundred dollars, so I told him about a drug company assistance program that he was eligible for. The patient reached for his phone, and, literally within minutes, he was able to register for the program. He saved hundreds of dollars instantly.

Chapter 12
What You Don't Know About Meds Can Hurt You

All About Medication Errors

Medication drug use—whether by prescription or purchased over-the-counter—is very common. In fact, a third of American adults use at least five or more medications routinely.[41] Preventing medication errors is an important issue, and the pharmacist takes it seriously.

A medication error occurs when a mistake on a prescription order gets to the patient. It can pertain to the drug itself, the dosage, or the amount. For example:

- Esomeprazole 40 mg was prescribed, but *Omeprazole* 40mg was dispensed.
- Furosemide 20mg was prescribed to be taken "every other day," but the pill bottle says "every day."
- Sixty tablets of Ibuprofen 800mg were prescribed, but there were only 30 tablets in the bottle.

Although medication errors are an unfortunate reality in the health care system, detecting and preventing a medication error before it gets to the patient is one of the many reasons the pharmacy profession exists today.

Every pharmacist dreads making an error on a prescription. But mistakes happen, and they are more likely to occur when they are rushed and distracted. Unfortunately, that is often the norm in the retail community pharmacy, where short-staffing runs rampant, and a single pharmacist is completing jobs that require a whole team of pharmacists. Some pharmacists work 10 to 12 hours a day with no scheduled breaks, dispensing hundreds of prescriptions a day. As previously discussed, pharmacists don't just process and dispense prescriptions; they are administering vaccinations and providing clinical services such as blood pressure checks, medication counseling, and consultations. Pharmacists are increasingly stepping up, trying to bridge the gap in patient health care; even so, they are sometimes marginalized by the industry they love. This has a negative effect on quality, and when quality suffers, errors occur, and patients may lose confidence in the health care system.

I support the continued expanded roles of pharmacists, but I wish that pharmacists would get the resources, staffing, and systems they need to fulfill these added roles. The reality is: on the front lines of community health care, they do not. Pharmacists nationwide are sounding an alarm and sharing their experiences about how staffing deficiencies are resulting in dangerous work environments that are becoming breeding ground for medication errors.[42]

As a health care provider, I strongly believe that there are no shortcuts to providing quality patient care. Patient care has to be done right each and every time.

When you suspect a medication error, the first thing to do is to notify the pharmacist as quickly as possible. If an error occurs on your medication, your pharmacist takes it seriously and will diligently work to resolve it. Call and ask to speak to the pharmacist or, if possible, return to the pharmacy and speak with them there.

Here are some simple, proactive steps you can take to minimize the issues with medication errors:

1. Always open and review the contents of your prescription bag before you leave the pharmacy.

2. Ask questions. You always want to know which medications you are getting before you pay. If, for any reason, you do not need any of the medications you've received, notify the pharmacist immediately.

3. Always notify the pharmacist when any of your medications change or are discontinued. Medications that your doctor has discontinued or changed will need to be deactivated so that they are not accidentally reordered in the future. This is especially important if you use automatic refill services to fulfill your medication order. If you don't deactivate them, they will likely keep being auto-refilled, and you may be charged for medicine you don't need or use.

4. Always keep a current list of your medications. If possible, memorize them. You could find it frustrating if you only refer to your blood pressure medicine as "the small, pink tablet." Know the names of the medicines you take, how you take them, and what you take them for.

5. Always request a consultation with the pharmacist for any medications that you are not familiar with or have questions about.

6. Always give specific instructions to the pharmacy when you turn in your prescriptions. Your doctor might write multiple medicines on one paper hardcopy. If you don't need them all filled at the time, notify the pharmacy right when you drop off the prescription. The pharmacist can dispense the ones you need and put a hold on the others that you don't need right away.

7. Don't rush the pharmacist. Give them adequate time to prepare your medicines.

8. Each time you turn in or pick up a prescription, you'll need to provide the patient's name and date of birth to help prevent errors. Don't assume the pharmacy knows who you are, even though they probably do. When you are picking up some medicine for someone other than yourself, you'll need to know the legal name and date of birth of the patient.

9. Since families often use the same pharmacy for their medication needs, when you pick up or drop off a prescription, let the pharmacy know if you are requesting medicines for just one person or multiple people. Give the first and last names and birthdates for all persons you are picking up for.

10. When you get home, and before you begin taking your medication, carefully read and review your pill bottle and the accompanying drug information materials. Ensure that your unique personal information, such as your name and date of birth, are correct. If you have any questions about your medications or if you need to clarify any discrepancies, call your pharmacist right away.

Adverse Reactions (Side effects)

Even when you get the proper medication care—the right drug, the right dose, the right duration at the right price—adverse reactions, or unwanted side effects of the medication, can still occur.

No matter how minor a prescription or over-the-counter drug is, it has the potential to cause an adverse reaction. Side effects can range from minor or moderate—such as nausea, upset stomach, bitter or metallic after-taste, hives, dizziness, insomnia, or cough—to major problems such as palpitation, respiratory problems, hypertension, tremors, or anaphylaxis. Minor to moderate side effects will often subside over time once your body has adjusted to your medicine. When you experience a drug side effect that continues to linger with no resolution, you should seek advice from your pharmacist and prescribing doctor. For severe life-threatening adverse reactions, such as anaphylactic shock, you should get emergency care immediately.

The inner workings of the body are as unique as your fingerprint. As a result, there is a lot of variability with each individual's response to a drug. One person might take a drug and experience little or no side effects, while another person can take the exact same medication and have a bad reaction to it. How the body processes and responds to a drug differs from person to person and will determine the side effect that is experienced.

Some contributing factors that can cause a patient to experience side effects can include:

- Age
- Higher dose
- Hypersensitivity and allergies
- Low or compromised immune system

- Slow metabolism
- Genetic predisposition and variability
- Compromised liver or kidney function

Common drug side effects [43]

- Antibiotics can cause stomach upset, diarrhea, hives.
- Antihistamines can cause drowsiness, dry mouth.
- Benzodiazepines can cause fatigue, sedation, low blood pressure, memory impairment.
- Cold/sinus medicines containing oral nasal decongestants can increase blood pressure, insomnia, restlessness, hyperactivity.
- Iron supplements can cause stomach cramping, constipation, urine discoloration, metallic taste.
- Narcotic pain medicines can cause constipation, respiratory depression, drowsiness.
- Oral nonsteroidal anti-inflammatory drugs (NSAIDs) can cause stomach pain, ulcers, nausea, indigestion.
- Orally inhaled steroids can cause oral thrush, increase blood glucose, headache, upper respiratory tract infection.
- Skeletal muscle relaxants can cause drowsiness, dry mouth, nausea.
- Steroids can cause insomnia, nervousness, high blood sugar, increased appetite.

When it comes to medications, it's important to remember that it's always possible for side effects to occur. Be aware of what side effects your medications might cause and make adjustments when you can. For example, if the medication you have been prescribed is known to cause an upset stomach, you should eat a meal prior to taking it. If the medication you have been prescribed is known to cause constipation, you should increase your daily dietary fiber while on the medication.

Your Medicine Isn't Ready? Here's Why.

As I've mentioned earlier, delays at the pharmacy are common—sometimes even necessary—as much as we might not like them. Unfortunately, many patients are more frustrated than they need to be because they don't understand some of the many factors that make it possible to get the medication they need at a pharmacy nearby.

Here are a few questions pharmacists hear a lot:

"But the pharmacist told me my medication would be ready at 2 p.m.! Why is it not done?"
"But my doctor told me to pick it up right away! Why isn't it ready?"
"But you told me my medication was ordered for today! So why isn't it here yet?"

If it helps, always remember that the pharmacist is your advocate and will work diligently to help you work around any issues that cause delays in receiving your medication.

Here's an in-depth look at the most common reasons for prescription delays:

• ***The prescription needs clarification or validation.***

Pharmacists sometimes need to contact a prescribing doctor to clarify or validate a medication order. All prescriptions undergo a validation process before the pharmacist can dispense them. If a prescription isn't validated, the pharmacist will notify the prescribing doctor, and the order will be placed on standby until the prescribing doctor supplies the necessary information to validate it. A prescription will typically fail the validation process if it is missing any of the following information: the medication's dose, formulation, quantity, instructions, issue date, provider-specific national provider number or drug enforcement agency number (for controlled substances), doctor's signature, or illegible handwritten prescription. When any of these prescription flaws occur, your prescription order will be delayed and cannot be legally dispensed until resolved.

• ***Your early refill is denied.***

Your insurance plan might deny your medication request because it is too soon to refill it, according to the last time it was filled. When this occurs, your prescription will be delayed, and the expected pick-up date will be determined by your insurance company.

For example, let's say you purchased 30 tablets of your blood pressure medication, Quinapril 20mg, on May 1 using your insurance plan. The medication order has you taking one tablet daily. But if you tried to get another refill on May 13, your insurance company would probably deny the claim because it is early. Since you picked up a 30-day supply on May 1, it was calculated that you shouldn't be out of the medication on the 13th. If you are taking the medication correctly, your supply should last you until May 31. Keeping track of early refills is one way the industry contains the cost of excessive health care spending and prevents waste and unnecessary duplication of treatments. Most insurance companies will give you a three-to-five-day early grace period from the last fill date of a non-controlled prescription. In this case, for example, the earliest fill date could be around May 26.

Quick Rx Tip: There are certain situations such as travel, lost/stolen medicines, or therapy changes that might justify an early medication refill. If this applies to your prescription, you should notify the pharmacist. The pharmacist can notify the insurance company of your special circumstances and request an exception for your situation.

- ***The prescription is not covered by the insurance company.***

Sometimes, your insurance will not cover a prescribed medication. This can happen if the medication prescribed by your doctor is a non-formulary drug or requires prior step therapy. To resolve this, your insurance company might require that your doctor provide additional information to support that the prescribed medication is medically necessary before your medication can be considered for coverage. Your doctor might also have to complete a prior authorization form provided by your insurance company. The entire prior authorization process can take as little as a few hours or as long as 14 days or more. Once your doctor has successfully submitted the prior authorization documentation, it is reviewed by the insurance company.

Once an insurance review process is complete, the insurance company will notify your doctor or pharmacy of their decision to approve or deny the medication in question. In cases where the insurance company denies a prior authorization request, they typically provide the reason for the medication denial and the criteria needed in order for an approval to occur. For example, your insurance company might require that you first use and have failed a less expensive drug before the plan will cover the more expensive one. The criterion is also known as a *prerequisite* or step therapy requirement.

Your insurance plan can also use clinical practice guidelines to determine what goes on the drug formulary. Clinical practice guidelines are science-based protocols that help doctors prescribe the most appropriate drugs for specific conditions.[44] If your insurance plan determines that your doctor might not be following the appropriate step therapy guidelines, they can require that the doctor submit a prior authorization form. When the prior authorization process is completed, your doctor or pharmacist will inform you of the result. If the medication in question is denied, you can choose to pay for the medication out-of-pocket, or the doctor can write a prescription for a different medication, one that is considered a preferred formulary alternative.

When the insurance company recommends or prefers a different drug, the pharmacist will notify the ordering physician. If the doctor decides to change the medication, a new prescription will be needed.

Keep in mind that your doctor or pharmacist might not know what is covered or not covered with your specific insurance plan. There is no uniformity of drug formularies across insurance plans; each insurance plan or group determines its own unique drug formulary using a pharmacy benefit management company. Likewise, just because one insurance plan covers a drug doesn't mean that it will be covered under a different insurance plan. This is especially significant for patients who change insurance plans from year to year. It's a common occurrence that a medication that a patient has been taking routinely for months or years gets denied, and the new insurance plan requires a prior authorization to be completed.

It is imperative for you as a patient to be proactive. If your pharmacist informs you that your medication is not ready due to the need for prior authorization, you should first notify your doctor and then take the initiative to contact your insurance company as well. Speaking directly with them is critical because you will receive the most in-depth information about why your medication is not covered, which alternative medications might be covered, and what options you might have to file an appeal.

Always remember to be an active participant in your health care decisions because it will save you time and money on your medications.

Here's a quick summary of what happens when a prior authorization is needed:

1. Your doctor writes a prescription.
2. The pharmacist receives the prescription and reviews it.
3. The pharmacist processes the prescription and bills the insurance company.
4. The insurance company rejects the prescription, requiring a prior authorization.
5. The pharmacist notifies the doctor that a prior authorization is needed.
6. The doctor's office routes the prior authorization request to the designated personnel.
7. The doctor contacts the insurance company, completes the necessary forms and documentation, and submits them to the insurance company.
8. The insurance company reviews the submitted documentation and either approves or denies the prescription.

9. The doctor's office notifies the pharmacist of approval or denial.

10. The pharmacist notifies the patient of the prior authorization results.

11. *If approved*, the pharmacist dispenses the prescription; you pay the insurance copay and receive your medicine.

12. *If denied*, you have a decision to make. You can choose to pay out-of-pocket for your medication, or you can request that the doctor change to a covered alternative.

> **Quick Rx Tip:** It's very important to remember that even though your doctor has given you a prescription, it doesn't necessarily mean that your insurance plan will automatically pay for it!

• ***Your medication isn't available.***

Sometimes a pharmacy might not have your medication available on the shelf. When this happens, the pharmacist will place an order for it. Depending on the availability from the drug distributor or drug manufacturer, it can take as quickly as the next day or as long as a few days for the ordered medication to arrive. If you need the medication urgently and you cannot wait, you can request that the pharmacy check with a different pharmacy to inquire if they have your medication available.

Even after the pharmacist has ordered it for you, the drug might not get shipped right away. This is because some drugs can become unavailable due to a manufacturer shortage, backorder, product discontinuation, or some other supply-chain issue. Supply issues are beyond the control of the pharmacist and can cause delays in your medication order.

• ***There's a drug shortage.***

Drug shortages are a common occurrence in the pharmacy industry and occur when a drug has limited availability or there is not enough medication to meet demand. Drug shortages can be a huge problem for outpatient and inpatient pharmacists as well as patients. In one year alone, up to 210 drugs have been in short supply.[45] Drug shortages can be caused by manufacturing production delays, manufacturing plant closures, shortage of raw materials, drug recalls, and inclement weather conditions that affect distribution.

> **Quick Rx Tip:** If you are unable to get your prescription due to a shortage issue, instead of waiting indefinitely, it might be best to contact your doctor and ask for a change in medication so there is no disruption in your medication therapy. Drug shortages are unpredictable and can take several days, weeks, or even months to resolve.

Wholesale distributors purchase drugs from drug manufacturers, which, in turn, supply the drugs to pharmacies. All it takes is some disruption in the supply chain, no matter how small, to affect the availability of the pills that go into your medication bottle.

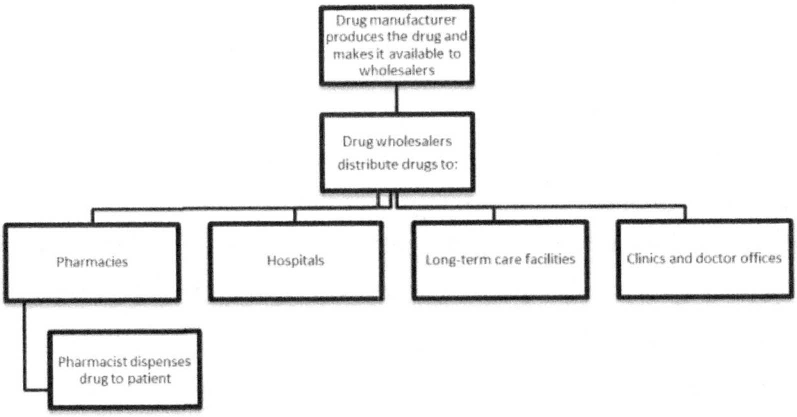

• ***The pharmacist can't supply your whole order right away.***

From time to time, you might receive a partial supply of your medicine because a pharmacy does not have the entire quantity of your medicine on hand. The pharmacist wants you to start your medication right away, so if they're short on supply, they might give you a few days' supply to get started and place an order for the balance of your medicine. But that can take a few days to arrive. When you receive a partial order, be sure to return to the pharmacy within a few days (usually three to five days) to get the rest of your medicine. It is a good idea to call ahead first to verify that the pharmacy has, in fact, received it. If you wait too long to pick up the balance of your medication, the order might be considered a "no show" and get returned.

If you have insurance, you will probably be charged a portion of your copay for the partial supply you received. When you return to pick up the rest of your medication order, your insurance will charge you the remaining copay. For example, let's say the full copay on your order is $20 for 30 tablets, but the pharmacist did not have 30 tablets of the medication in stock. So, to get you started, they give you a partial order of six tablets. Your insurance might charge you $5 for a partial fill of six tablets, and when you pick up the balance of 24 tablets, you will pay the balance of $15.

$5 + $15= $20 (total copay)

When you are using insurance, your pharmacist does not determine your copayment costs; your insurance company does. Your insurance company might charge you the full copay on your partial supply. For example, if your copay is $5 for 60 tablets, and you only pick up a partial order of 10 tablets, you might have to pay the $5. When you pick up the rest of your medicine, the copay will be zero.

$5 + $0= $5 (total copay)

If you don't have insurance, your price will be calculated based on the quantity you are receiving.

Quick Rx Tip: When your medication order is filled, pick it up as soon as possible. Find out your pharmacy's policy about how long you have to pick up a scheduled medication. Once processed, the pharmacist will keep your medicines ready for you for a week or two. If you do not pick up within the allotted time, your medication might be returned back to inventory.

• ***Pharmacies are open to the public and anyone can consult with the pharmacist. Anytime. For free.***

Community pharmacies generally have an open-door policy and are open to anyone who needs to consult with a pharmacist, even without an appointment. This simple fact can make the patient pharmacy experience and wait times unpredictable for both walk-in and over-the-phone patient consultations.

You can literally walk into the pharmacy and get a professional consultation from the pharmacist, and you pay—what? Zero. Nada. Zilch. Zip. Absolutely nothing. This is one of the most unique and extraordinary things about community pharmacists. With high health care costs, patients are increasingly turning to their local neighborhood pharmacists for health care advice and information. The pharmacist's accessibility is one of the reasons why we are pulled in a hundred different directions and why, no matter how hard or how fast we work, your prescriptions might not be ready at the time you expected.

• ***Pharmacies are taking shortcuts.***

Can you imagine a pilot operating a passenger airplane without flight attendants? Or a medical doctor practicing without nurses? A pharmacist, too, cannot practice without adequate support personnel. In my 20-plus years in the pharmaceutical care industry, one simple fact has held true: There are no shortcuts to caring for patients. Caring for patients is an extremely rewarding yet time-intensive job. The unfortunate reality is that many pharmacy health care businesses do take shortcuts under the guise of cutting costs and saving money. Quite often, these shortcuts leave pharmacies understaffed and underequipped, compromising the quality and the integrity of the pharmacist-patient relationship. Imagine if a pilot had to check-in and board passengers, attend to the needs of the passengers, and fly the plane, too! It would be mayhem! Pharmacists in retail community pharmacies around the country are doing the equivalent of that. Because of this, delays will occur.

More Tips About Medications

- Take your medicine and follow your doctor's orders. Adherence is essential to your health. The medicine cannot work if you don't take it.
- Do not make any assumptions about how to take your medicine. Read your pill bottle and the prescription information attached before you take it. Call the pharmacist for any questions or concerns.
- Be an informed patient. Do your research but be careful not to fall down the self-diagnosis rabbit hole based on information you found on TV or the internet. Always go see a doctor or medical professional for a proper consult and diagnosis. Because a television guru or social media star endorses a medication does not imply it's safe or healthy for you.

- If you have somewhat complicated issues about your medicine in the pharmacy and are confused about what to do next, you can simply ask to speak to the pharmacist. The pharmacist can consult with you and your doctor to address your medication concerns.
- You cannot return a prescription medication just because you changed your mind and decide you don't want it anymore. Buyer's remorse is real, so prior to paying for your medication, you want to be 100% certain about your purchase. Once you have purchased a prescription medicine and left the pharmacy, it cannot be returned unless there is an extenuating reason, such as a medication error. When a medication error occurs, the medicine is quarantined and disposed of; it cannot be reused or resold.
- When it comes to drug information, you will be very frustrated if you take the word of anyone other than your pharmacist. Your coworker, family member, and even your doctor don't have the most up-to-date information on drug pricing and inquiries.
- If you are told your medicine is on backorder, here's what you should know. A medication backorder simply means that the medication that's been ordered for you is having a supply issue and might not be available yet. Drug supply issues occur for a variety of reasons. For example, a manufacturer might discontinue production, there might be a limited supply at the manufacturer due to things like a shortage of ingredients, and delays at the distribution level, such as transportation and weather-related issues.
- Sometimes the look and feel of medications change. When there have been no changes to your prescription, but the pill itself has a different shape, color, or size, it usually means

the pharmacist is using a different drug manufacturer for the medication. The pharmacy receives medication from multiple drug manufacturers due to market supply and demand. The physical appearance of bioequivalent generic medicines that are made by different manufacturing companies might not be the same. For example:

Losartan 100mg is a medication used to treat high blood pressure. Different generic drug manufacturing companies make it. When made by Teva, it is a green, oblong pill with imprint 93 and 7366. If made by Aurobindo, it is a green, oval pill with imprint E and 47. If made by Apotex, it is a round white pill with imprint APO and LS 100. If made by Actavis, it is a green oval pill with imprint LK 100.

Amoxicillin 500mg is another example. When made by Sandoz, the capsule is yellow with imprint GG and 849. When made by Teva, it is brown with imprint 3109. When made by Dava, it is pink and red with imprint WC and 731. Made by Northstar, it is blue and pink with imprint A45. If it is manufactured by Westward, then it is white with imprints westward and 939.

- Manufacturers of generic medications cannot make them look identical because it is a violation of copyright. The pharmacist will notify you verbally or use a label or handwritten note on your bag when this occurs. Drug manufacturer changes on medications are a common occurrence that are beyond the control of the pharmacist. So, don't panic if there is a drug manufacturer change on your medication. You can always call the pharmacist to verify if you have any questions.

- Some pharmacies cannot dispose of used medications. By law, pharmacies cannot take medications back for disposal unless they are a registered, authorized prescription disposal site with the Drug Enforcement Agency (DEA)—and not all are. To find a registered disposal site near you, visit the DEA website at www.dea.gov. A pharmacy that is a registered disposal site will usually have a self-service kiosk where you can safely and discreetly dispose of your unwanted medications. You can also dispose of medications during community prescription take-back events that are hosted by the fire department or local DEA office. These events will usually be advertised in your community.
- Sometimes people take the wrong pill by mistake. It is becoming all too common because more people are using pill organizers and combining different medicines in one organizer, which can sometimes lead to confusion and medication mix-ups. Unless you have extenuating circumstances, it is safer to keep your medications in their original container. If pill organizers aren't carefully refilled, you might take one pill when you intended to take a different one. When this happens, you should immediately call your pharmacist or health care provider.
- If you accidentally take a double dose of your medicine, you might need to skip the next dose of the medicine. To be safe, call your pharmacist or health care provider as soon as possible.
- If you forgot to take your medication, take it as soon as possible after a missed dose. If it is already time for your next dose, you should not take a double dose unless told to do so by your health care provider. Call your pharmacist or health care provider for advice.

- If you have been taking your medication as prescribed, but you don't feel your medication is working, don't abruptly stop it unless you are having an allergic reaction to it. Some medications can take up to a few days or weeks before you begin to feel the full effects or response. Discuss your concerns with your doctor or pharmacist.
- If you think you're having an allergic reaction to a medicine, notify your doctor immediately. If you have a mild allergic reaction to a medicine, for example, a minor rash or hives, you might be able to use an antihistamine called diphenhydramine to help soothe the allergic reaction. If you are having a serious anaphylactic reaction such as a blistering rash, difficulty breathing, and shortness of breath, or if you feel your throat tighten up, you should seek emergency care immediately by calling 911. People who have serious, life-threatening allergies should talk to their doctor about getting Epinephrine on hand to use for severe allergic reactions. Epinephrine is available by prescription in an automated intramuscular pen injection that can be used to stop a serious allergic reaction when an emergency occurs.
- Do not take expired medications. Regardless of whether a drug expired three days, one month, or six months ago, expired medications should be disposed of and not be consumed because the quality, potency, and safety could be compromised.
- Changes to prescriptions sometimes take time. A prescription is a legal document, and any changes to it, such as drug, dose, or quantity, require authorization from the prescribing doctor. By law, if any change to the prescription is required, your doctor will be contacted, but

no changes can be made without the doctor's knowledge and approval.

- To prevent delays with your prescriptions, make a habit of asking your doctor to write you a new prescription if the instructions on your prescription bottle or hardcopy prescription are different from your doctor's verbal instructions. The pharmacist can only dispense your prescription as legally written. For example, let's say you've been taking your diabetes medication once a day, but at your last office visit, your doctor said she wanted you to increase the dose to twice a day. In that case, your doctor should give you a brand-new prescription with the new dose because you will run out of medicine sooner if you are taking it more often. Although you might still have available refills on record, your insurance company might not pay for the refill because the doctor did not issue a new prescription with the increased dose.

About Controlled Medications

What is a controlled substance, and why does it always seem like it's a hassle to get prescriptions for controlled substances filled? A controlled substance is a medication that is regulated by law due to the risks of abuse and dependency.

There are five classes of controlled substances based on the risk of abuse and dependency. Class 1 has the highest risk, and Class 5 has the lowest risk, as follows:[46]

- Class 1: These are known as illicit drugs. They have a high level of abuse and are the only class of controlled substances that have no legal medical use. For example, heroin and cocaine.

- Class 2: These drugs have a high risk of abuse and dependency. They can be used for the treatment of pain and include medications like morphine, hydrocodone, oxycodone, fentanyl, hydromorphone, and methadone. They can also be used in the treatment of Attention Deficit Hyperactive Disorder (ADHD) and include medications like Concerta, Ritalin, Vyvanse, and Adderall.

- Class 3: These drugs have a low-to-moderate risk of abuse and dependency. For example: Tylenol with codeine, which is used for pain, and testosterone, which is used for hormone replacement.

- Class 4: These drugs have a lower risk of abuse and dependency. They include benzodiazepines, such as Alprazolam, Clonazepam, Lorazepam, Triazolam, and Diazepam; sleep medications, such as Ambien, Lunesta, and Sonata; and muscle relaxants, such as Soma.

- Class 5: These drugs have the lowest risk of abuse and dependency. They include medications like Lyrica, which is used for fibromyalgia, Lomotil, which is used for diarrhea, and Robitussin with Codeine, used for cough and cold symptoms.

Controlled substances are regulated by the Drug Enforcement Agency (DEA). Pharmacists are required by law to follow all state and federal laws when it comes to the dispensing of these medications. You need to have valid identification when presenting or picking up a prescription for a controlled substance.

A prescription for a controlled substance must contain the patient's information and the doctor's information, including their DEA number. The prescription needs to be written on a tamper-resistant paper and must be signed and dated by the doctor.

If a prescription for a controlled substance is missing some of the required information when presented to the pharmacist, it cannot be dispensed. The pharmacist has to follow the law; there is no room for noncompliance.

Class 2 controlled substances, such as hydrocodone, oxycodone, methadone, dextroamphetamine, fentanyl, and methylphenidate are the highest level of controlled substances for legitimate medical use.

Class 2 controlled substances cannot be transferred between pharmacies. For example, let's say your doctor's office sends an Electronic Class 2 controlled prescription for Vyvanse to Pharmacy A for you. However, if you realized you couldn't make it to Pharmacy A, and you want to pick it up at Pharmacy B, your doctor would have to cancel the order at Pharmacy A and resend it to Pharmacy B since it is non-transferable. Or, say that you turned in your hardcopy prescription for your medication of hydromorphone to Pharmacy C, but you find out that Pharmacy C doesn't have the medication available. So, you decide you want to use Pharmacy D, which has the medication available. To do that, you would have to take your hardcopy prescription from Pharmacy C and physically turn it in to Pharmacy D in order to get your prescription filled.

When Your Medications Change

Every year, nearly 35 million people have health care needs that lead to an inpatient hospital admission, and millions more receive treatment from outpatient facilities.[47] Whether it's an inpatient or outpatient stay, you or your caregiver will be asked to provide a list of your current medications and dosage. Making sure you provide accurate and complete medication history is critical to your care.

A health emergency can occur at any time, so always carry a list of your current medications with you in a wallet or organizer for easy access. Also, have the contact information of your pharmacy or pharmacies so that, if an emergency occurs, your pharmacist can be reached to verify your current medication regimen.

During your stay in a health care facility, you will be under the care of a team of health care providers that work together to coordinate your care. When you are discharged and released from the hospital, your medication regimen might change. You should be given a medication reconciliation form and a member of your care team should review it with you.

A Medication Reconciliation Form does exactly what the name implies —it reconciles all of your current medicines. It is one of the most important documents you have as you transition back to your home or to another health care facility. It lists in detail the medications you are to start, discontinue, or continue taking and gives you a summary of your treatment plan. After you are discharged, you might be given special instructions, for example, to schedule a follow-up appointment with a specialist or primary care provider, complete laboratory testing, or complete other needed procedures and documents to ensure the continuity of your care. It is critical to your care and recovery that you follow your discharge instructions, and it also reduces the risk of medication errors and of your need to be readmitted to the hospital. Be sure to bring your medication reconciliation list to your next follow-up visit with your doctor.

It is also a good idea to bring a copy of your Medication Reconciliation Form, along with your prescriptions, when you go to the pharmacy. The pharmacist can use the form to update your medication history and deactivate any old prescriptions that you shouldn't be taking anymore. The pharmacist can also help you interpret your medication reconciliation form so that you fully understand your treatment plan.

Sample Medication Reconciliation Form

Your Medications Have Changed

Current as of: December 13, 2021

Patient: Jane Doe

Patient Date of Birth: 5/25/1983

New Medication: Start taking Labetalol 300mg. Take 1 tablet by mouth every 8 hours. (Dose increased)

Medications to Continue: Prenatal vitamins: Take 1 tablet by mouth every day.

Medications to Stop: Ibuprofen 400mg and Labetalol 200mg

Reviewed by: John Doe, MD

If you have ever been admitted to the hospital, visited the doctor's office, had to go to the emergency room or even visited a pharmacy, you know firsthand that our health care system can seem fragmented and disconnected at times. A lot of improvement is still needed with health care system integration and coordination. Patients often see different health care providers who might be unaware of other tests or medicines that are being issued. This is why both patients and their health care providers have to be proactive to make sure that they have up-to-date health records.

Patients who have had a change or transition in care are especially vulnerable to errors, which is why caregivers and health care providers need to be especially vigilant with them to ensure there are no lapses in their continuity of care. This includes:

- Patients transitioning from a hospital to hospice care, nursing home, assisted living facility or moving to another facility.
- Patients transitioning from a hospital or other health care facility to their home.

Chapter 13
Crisis: Narcotics in America

America's consumption of pain medicines has become one of today's most alarming trends. The United States leads the world in demand for narcotic pain medications.

Opioids are a class of drugs that are used primarily to treat pain. They work by binding to opioid receptors in the body and brain, blocking pain signals, so even though the pain is there, you do not feel it. When opioids get into the body, the brain also releases dopamine, a neurotransmitter that activates the reward and pleasure system in the brain. The brain naturally releases dopamine in response to pleasurable stimulation from activities such as eating, having sex, and listening to music.[48]

The brain's reward-and-pleasure system encourages the body to do things that have a healthy, positive effect on the body, making it easy for them to become habitual.[49] But with exposure to opioid drugs, the body gets an artificial stimulation, which still causes the release of dopamine, generating a feeling of euphoria. And the continual use of opioids disrupts the body's natural system of dopamine release. With long-term exposure to opioid drugs, the body builds up a tolerance to it and, over time, it takes more and more of the drug to deliver the same effect. This can lead to a vicious cycle of chemical dependency and addiction.

Americans make up 5% of the world population but consume an astonishing 80% of the world's supply of pain medication. Because of the overuse and overprescribing of powerful opioid pain medicines, the number of people who die from prescription pain medicines now exceeds deaths from heroin and cocaine combined.[50]

Did You Know?

- Americans consume 56% of the world's supply of morphine.[51] Morphine is a drug used to treat pain and is classified as a Class 2 narcotic medication.
- Americans consume over 99% of the world's supply of hydrocodone.[52] Hydrocodone is the most commonly prescribed narcotic pain medicine. It is classified as a Class 2 narcotic medication and is available in combination with products such as acetaminophen and ibuprofen.
- Americans consume 81% of the world's supply of oxycodone.[53] Oxycodone is a Class 2 narcotic drug used to treat pain.
- Americans consume 43% of the global production of Fentanyl, one of the most lethal drugs in the United States.[54] A Class 2 narcotic drug, Fentanyl is used to treat pain. It is extremely potent and is the most common drug found in drug overdoses.[55]
- Americans consume 44% of the global production of methadone, a Class 2 narcotic drug used to treat pain.[56]
- Eight out of ten of the most common substances involved in overdose deaths are prescription drugs.
- The top ten drugs involved in overdose deaths are:
  1. Fentanyl: a narcotic pain medicine
  2. Heroin: an illegal substance with no medical use

3. Hydrocodone: a narcotic pain medicine
4. Methadone: a narcotic pain medicine
5. Morphine: a narcotic pain medicine
6. Oxycodone: a narcotic pain medicine
7. Alprazolam: a benzodiazepine used in the treatment of anxiety, panic disorder, and other conditions
8. Diazepam: a benzodiazepine used in the treatment of anxiety, panic disorder, and other conditions
9. Cocaine: an illegal substance with no medical use
10. Methamphetamine: a stimulant used in the treatment of Attention Deficit Hyperactivity Disorder (ADHD)

Other prescription drugs linked to overdose deaths include:

- Diphenhydramine: an antihistamine commonly found in cough and cold products
- Acetaminophen: a common ingredient in over-the-counter and prescription pain medicines
- Gabapentin: an anticonvulsant that can be used to treat pain
- Citalopram: an antidepressant used to treat depression
- Tramadol: used to treat pain
- Amitriptyline: an antidepressant used to treat depression
- Oxymorphone: a narcotic pain medicine
- Clonazepam: a benzodiazepine used in the treatment of seizures, panic disorder, and other conditions

The epidemic of opioid abuse disorder is devastating communities and has finally begun to make national headlines. So that history does not repeat itself, we need to ask ourselves how we got here. The crisis did not happen overnight. A long history of flawed pain management guidelines and policy initiatives, aggressive marketing and distribution by drug manufacturers, overprescribing, inadequate regulatory oversight of the approval, production, marketing, and distribution of narcotic drugs has led us to this breaking point.

The Opioid Crisis

The Veteran Affairs Health System, the largest integrated health care system in the United States, is funded by the federal government and sets policy standards that other health systems across the country model and use. In 1999, it promoted a policy of treating pain as a fifth vital sign.[57] The policy recommended that pain assessment be addressed at every encounter with a patient, and it tied pain assessment to patient satisfaction surveys.[58] Subsequently, many other health systems and medical associations across the country adopted the policy and integrated it into their protocols. In response, clinicians, recognizing patient pain assessment scores were tied to patient satisfaction surveys—which affect hospital reimbursements—began overprescribing opioids. They were also motivated to avoid the dreaded malpractice claim.[59]

For the nearly two decades that the U.S. health care system treated pain as the fifth vital sign, prescription pill mills took it as a license to prescribe pain medication cocktails. They were left unchecked as they pumped patients and communities with medically unnecessary narcotic drugs that were being abused, misused, and diverted. In many local communities, regulatory and law enforcement agencies did not have the logistical capacity to address such a complex problem at the different levels it manifested and were unable to mitigate the problem.

Simultaneously, drug companies were heavily marketing narcotic pain medications even as they downplayed their risk of dependency and addiction. For a long time, billboards and other signs advertising pain management clinics on the roadsides and highways were everywhere. There were clinics in strip malls that had providers who would write a prescription for any controlled narcotic substance of the patient's choice, feeding patients addiction. Before long, powerful prescription narcotic drugs were being prescribed irresponsibly, their use was treated too casually, and they became the drugs of choice for far too many for both acute and chronic pain.

True Story

While at work years ago, I received a phone call from a physician calling in a verbal prescription for a narcotic pain medication. While we casually chatted, he told me that he was a retired doctor calling in a prescription for his neighbor. He was just doing a favor, he said. Red flags began to go off in my head. I asked if there was a patient-doctor relationship, and he said there wasn't. The doctor told me his DEA license was still active, and that gave him the authority to prescribe a narcotic medication. He admitted that he hadn't examined the neighbor.

I informed him that, as a pharmacist, I had a responsibility to ensure that this narcotic prescription was being prescribed based upon a patient-doctor relationship after examining the patient. But, based on the information he had given me, I could not in good conscience dispense the prescription.

He was upset. He asserted his rights as a doctor, which I politely acknowledged, but I also reminded him that as a pharmacist, I too have corresponding rights and must abide by the oath and laws that govern my profession. He asked for my name and license information, which I gave him.

I took the liberty of calling the neighbor "patient", explaining why I could not dispense the prescription in good faith. I suggested other over-the-counter options that were available and referred him to a primary care physician and the closest urgent care facility. The individual was gracious, understood my reservations, and thanked me for the courtesy call.

A few weeks later, I got a visit from my state's Board of Pharmacy. The agent explained that the physician in question had filed a complaint against me for declining to dispense the narcotic prescription he called in. I explained the reasons for my actions, and the agent reaffirmed that ethically and professionally, I had done the right and lawful thing.

As a pharmacist, my job is to protect patients from harm, even concerns they don't realize are there or may not understand.

~~~

Finally, in 2016, almost 20 years after the policy was introduced, and in response to the overwhelming opioid abuse crisis, the American Medical Association (AMA) finally recommended discontinuing the practice of promoting pain as the fifth vital sign.

To be able to answer my earlier question of how this opioid crisis has gotten so bad, it's important to recognize that the casual mis-prescribing of opioid medications that went unchecked is partly to blame. Truth be told, all of us health care providers—clinicians, doctors, pharmacists, nurses, health care administrators, and policy stakeholders—must examine our own practices and ask the tough questions. How did we contribute to the problem? How did this happen on our watch? The hard truth is that this did not simply happen overnight; it has taken us several years to get to where it is now. Real solutions are needed to tackle this growing health hazard.
~~~

Manufacturers marketed their potent narcotic pain medications as having a low risk of addiction, and it played a big role in their popularity. We now know that claim is false. Doctors were encouraged to prescribe more and more opioids to treat pain. More was considered better. Many patients were titrated to large doses of narcotic drugs, and their bodies naturally built up a tolerance to the high doses. Patients eventually found it difficult to stop taking the drugs.

The circumstances created a vicious cycle. A patient gets prescribed a pain medicine after an injury, dental work, surgery, or medical procedure. While under the care of a doctor, they were taking legally prescribed pain medication and eventually get hooked and chemically dependent on them. After their providers stop writing prescriptions for them, patients still want more drugs and turn to pill mills or the black market to get them. Getting drugs from the black market is a dangerous last resort that some patients turn to. It can be deadly because many street drugs are laced with other dangerous drugs and chemicals unknown to the patient.

The process leads to a cycle of abuse, overdose, and sometimes death. And it affects people of all kinds—students, athletes, professionals, young, old, male, female—you name it.

Pill Mills

Truthfully, I saw this storm coming many years ago. When I began my career as a pharmacist in 2007, I was shocked by what I saw on the front lines of community practice in Georgia. Narcotic pill mills were out of control, prescribing astonishing amounts of narcotic medications and popping up everywhere, often in affluent suburban areas. A prescription pill mill is a medical practice that claims to be a pain management clinic but is actually pushing narcotics pills, profiting from the addictions and drug diversions of their patients. Patients at these facilities don't receive proper medical care, physical examination, medical history evaluation, or diagnostic tests. They tell the doctor what drugs they want, and the doctor prescribes them. In 2007, I witnessed pill mill doctors prescribing astonishingly large quantities of narcotic drugs such as methadone, oxycodone, morphine, hydromorphone, hydrocodone, carisoprodol, and alprazolam for no legitimate medical need. I remember seeing advertising signs and flyers from "designer" pain clinics at corner stops, gas stations, shopping centers, on the roadside, and on highways.

For example, a person came into the pharmacy with prescriptions for:

- Norco 10/235mg #180
- Oxycodone 30mg #120
- Xanax 2mg #180
- Soma 350mg #120

All for one patient!

As a community pharmacist, I witness this every day. I see patients coming in with multiple prescriptions for large quantities of narcotic medications from prescription pill mills. Every day, patients trickle in, back-to-back, with identical drug cocktails from the same doctor. I call the doctor's office to verify the authenticity of the prescriptions and to find out the medical diagnosis that warranted their use. I don't get a logical answer. When I ask to speak to the doctor, I'm told that the doctor is unavailable, and my request for a call back does not get returned.

As a pharmacist trained in pain management, when I raise clinical concerns and a provider blatantly disregards them or chooses not to address them—and in so doing endangers the life or health of a patient—then I have a responsibility to the patient to ensure their safety. To do that, I must refuse to dispense a prescription that could cause harm. I exercise that legal recourse and continue to do so, despite receiving threats. During the same time period, there was a rise in pharmacy robberies, and sometimes, pharmacists were held up at gunpoint for narcotic drugs. It was a frightening time for my peers and me.

The overprescribing of narcotic drugs in my community was getting out of control. Finally, I felt that I had had enough, and I decided to canvas the pill mills to get more insight into their practices and then report them to law enforcement. I found out that many of these local "clinics" did not accept third-party insurance and were cash-only clinics. Patients would pay $300 to $500 cash per visit and walk out with large amounts of narcotic prescriptions. Their parking lots were full of cars with out-of-state license plates, a sign that they were fueling drug trafficking across state lines. Apparently, the news was out on the streets that the neighborhood pill mills in Georgia were open for business.

With the information I gathered, I cried foul. I reported the pill mills to law enforcement, but that didn't seem to stop the practice. One pill mill would close, only to pop up at another location under a different clinic name. The cycle continued for years despite my having alerted law enforcement.

Here's an excerpt of a letter I wrote to the DEA about it:

June 22, 2011
Drug Enforcement Agency
Diversion Control, Atlanta Division
Hello, my name is Dr. Yemi Brown. I am a staff pharmacist. I am writing to express concern regarding area pain clinics that I believe are over-prescribing highly addictive control medications. These pain clinics are writing prescriptions for medications such as oxycodone, Percocet, Xanax, Klonopin, and methadone in excessive quantities to patients that I believe are abusing and or diverting these drugs. It is my professional opinion that these clinics are operating pill mills. I am highly concerned that these pain clinics are engaged in unethical and illegal prescribing practices. Many of the patients coming from these clinics are being prescribed the same highly addictive drugs every 21 to 30 days, like clockwork. With the growing rate of accidental overdose from controlled substances, these pill mills are a huge detriment to our community and will continue to be a problem unless they are shut down promptly. I request and hope that you mount an official investigation. Do not hesitate to contact me for any assistance.

Sincerely,

Yemi Brown, PharmD

It blows my mind how my letter foreshadowed the opioid epidemic we are seeing today. I got a follow-up call and an on-site visit from a DEA agent, in which I provided all the information I had gathered. Unfortunately, I didn't see any immediate change as a result. The pill mills still continued their unethical and illegal practices.

Tracking the Problem

To truly understand the extent of the opioid prescription problem, we must look at the numbers and follow the trail of pills from manufacturer to consumer. One of the key tools the DEA has is its Automation of Reports and Consolidated Orders System (ARCOS), a system that tracks the manufacturing, distribution, and sale of controlled substances.[60] Data from the ARCOS has not previously been available publicly; however, a court ruling in 2019 allowed for the release to the public of ARCOS data from 2006 to 2012. Data from these records show that within a seven-year period, drug manufacturers flooded the U.S. market with 76 billion opioid pills. Oxycodone and hydrocodone made up 75% of those 76 billion pills.[61]

As the DEA had access to all that data already, though, it begs the question—what did the agency do with it? And should it have done more? While the opioid epidemic was escalating, the DEA's efforts to go after corrupt doctors, pharmacies, and providers that were affiliated with pill mills funneling opioid prescriptions to patients and the black market was slow and was not curbing the problem. Records show that the DEA took a bold step; it appealed directly to the main source—drug manufacturers and distributors—to slow down the production and distribution of opioid drugs by at least 30 to 40%. But the agency's requests were largely rejected or ignored.[62]

Over the past decade, the DEA has brought civil charges against several companies relating to the opioid crisis. These companies have paid fines totaling close to $500 million.[63]

In 2019, The Washington Post and HD Media won a lawsuit, giving it public access to the DEA ARCOS database.[64] The data revealed the following:

10 Top Distributors of Opioid Medications 2006 to 2012

1. McKesson Corporation	14,107,192,480 pills	18.4%
2. Walgreens	12,636,815,170 pills	16.5%
3. Cardinal Health	10,709,959,627 pills	14%
4. AmerisourceBergen	8,952,844,625 pills	11.7%
5. CVS	5,909,410,160 pills	7.7%
6. Walmart	5,255,663,660 pills	6.9%
7. Smith Drug Company	1,348,619,950 pills	1.8%
8. Rite Aid	1,314,386,010 pills	1.7%
9. Kroger	1,231,379,170 pills	1.6%
10. H. D. Smith	1,142,193,715 pills	1.5%

10 Top Manufacturers of Opioid Medications 2006 to 2012

1. SpecGx (a subsidiary of Mallinckrodt)	28,863,435,081 pills	37.7%
2. Actavis Pharma	26,476,395,830 pills	34.6%
3. Par Pharmaceutical	11,996,780,871 pills	15.7%
4. Purdue Pharma	2,492,496,319 pills	3.3%
5. Amneal Pharmaceutical	2,257,973,121 pills	2.9%
6. Teva Pharmaceutical USA	686,276,053 pills	0.9%
7. KVK Tech	580,825,207 pills	0.8%

8. Westward Pharmaceutical	384,200,988 pills	0.5%
9. Kaiser Foundation Hospitals	366,492,050 pills	0.5%
10. Endo Pharmaceuticals	297,306,324 pills	0.4%

How can it be that in just seven years, an astronomical number of opioid pills was pumped into communities across America? Advocates for the drug industry would say that they were providing opioid medications to legitimate patients with valid prescriptions who needed them. However, the reality is that these were extremely excessive amounts of opioid pills, they were not medically necessary, and they were getting funneled into the black market. They were being abused by legitimate patients due to the highly addictive and high chemical dependency of such powerful drugs. A patient using an opioid pill prescribed legitimately could easily become chemically dependent and addicted even if they took the pills correctly as prescribed by their doctor. Between 1999 and 2017, approximately 400,000 people lost their lives due to opioid overdose.[65]

Opioid Overdose Deaths —1999 to 2017

During this time, the number of opioid deaths steadily increased each year.

2017	47,600
2016	42,249
2015	33,091
2014	28,647
2013	25,052
2012	23,157
2011	22,784

2010	21,089
2009	20,422
2008	19,582
2007	18,516
2006	17,541
2005	14,910
2004	13,756
2003	12,940
2002	11,913
2001	9,496
2000	8,407
1999	8,050
Total opioid deaths	**399,202**[66]

Here are some more statistics:

- More people die from prescription overdoses than from heroin and cocaine combined.[67]
- As many as 15,000 people die annually from prescription overdose.[68]
- The highest number recorded to date is in 2017, when about 47,000 people died from prescription overdose.[69]
- The mortality rate of opioid overdose has increased steadily since the 90s. The persistent mortality rate of overdose deaths, especially in young adults, has contributed to a drop in total life expectancy.[70]

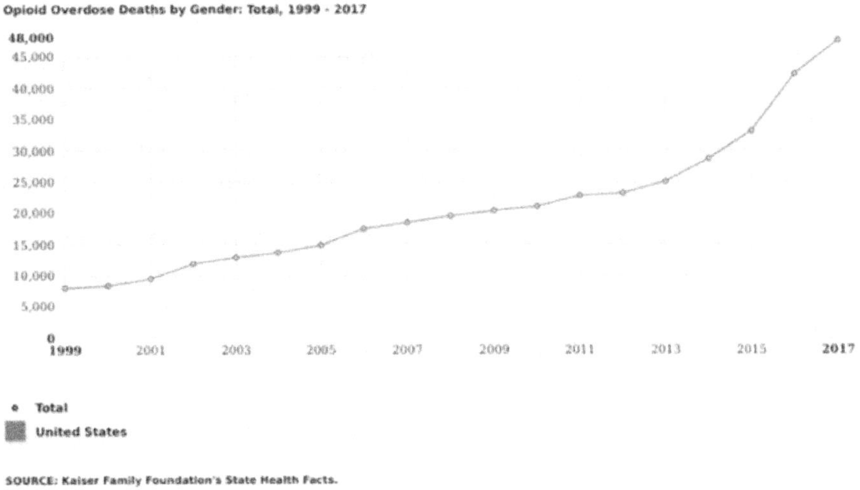

Deaths as a result of opioids make up the largest percentage of deaths relating to drug abuse overdose. The number has increased gradually from 48% in 1999 to 68% in 2017.[71]

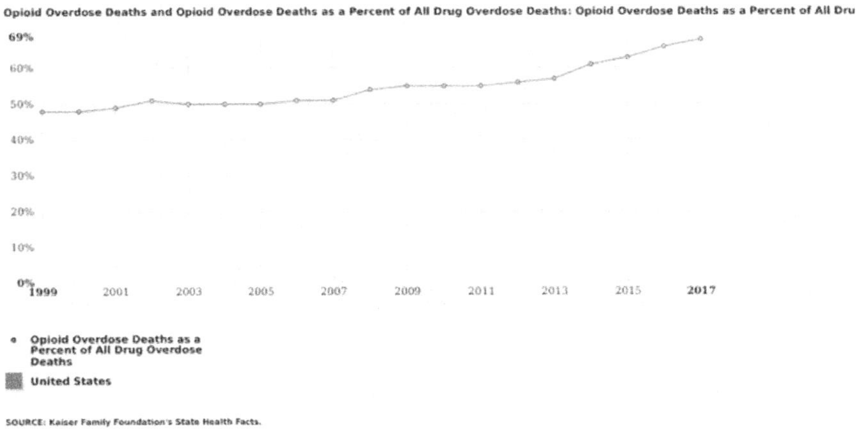

If you want to know how the opioid crisis has affected your state or local community, *The Washington Post* provides an extensive interactive site where you can find detailed information about how your state and local county has been affected.[72] Visit their website (www.WashingtonPost.com) and search for "DEA pain pill database" in the search menu.

More recently, many U.S. states are beginning to tackle the problem and are fighting back and going after health care providers that are involved with pill mills. Alabama, Georgia, Michigan, Texas, Tennessee, and Nevada are a few states that have found health care providers criminally liable for profiting from corrupt pill mill operations. In many cases, the clinics rake in millions of dollars at the expense of feeding many people's dangerous addictions.

Some states are also going after the main source of the problem—drug manufacturers. In the same way that Big Tobacco's feet were eventually held to the fire over the sale of cancer-causing cigarettes, Big Pharma should be held accountable, too. Slowly, they are. There are over 2,000 class-action lawsuits across counties in America, litigation against drug manufacturers for their culpability in fueling the opioid epidemic that has cost hundreds of thousands of lives and has left millions with opioid addiction.[73] States have also gone after drug distributors and pharmacies for their roles in the crisis too. Lawsuits against top manufacturers of opioid drugs are yielding billions of dollars in settlements.

In October 2020, the United States Justice Department reached a settlement with Purdue Pharma, the drug company that makes the pain medication Oxycontin. Purdue Pharma pleaded guilty to federal criminal charges that include conspiracy to defraud the U. S. government through deception and misrepresentation.[74] The drug company also pleaded guilty to violating the Food, Drug and Cosmetic Act and federal anti-kickback laws by promoting drug sales for illegitimate medical use and providing financial incentives to doctors who overprescribed their drug products.[75] Purdue Pharma will be fined over $8 billion.[76] It is yet to be seen how settlements like this one will be dispersed to state and local communities affected by opioid drug abuse.

There is plenty of finger-pointing about who is to blame for the epidemic. Is it the doctors' fault for writing prescriptions for large amounts of narcotics for patients? Or the drug companies for their unethical marketing practices? Or distributors that recklessly supplied the drugs? Or pharmacies and pharmacists that dispense the drugs to patients? Or the patient who knowingly or unknowingly mismanages these powerful medicines? Irrespective of who you think is to blame, it is undeniable that any health care system that could allow this to happen and fester for so long is failing badly. It is a reminder that a health care system that is primarily based on a for-profit model and that is allowed to go unregulated and unchecked is not in the best interest of patients collectively. It is a reminder that as a patient, you cannot blindly follow orders; you must have an active role in your care. Doing your research and asking questions about your care and treatment is essential to your health and safety.

Another problem that has fueled the pain pill addiction epidemic is the fact that for many years, patients did not have a hassle-free, safe, and effective way to dispose of unused or expired drugs such as pain medications.

Prior to 2014, pharmacies could not take back narcotic medications for disposal from the public. The rules have been relaxed a bit since then, partly due to the opioid epidemic. Recently, I've begun to see more pharmacies offering prescription disposal kiosks for patients. This is a big step forward.

Where do we go from here, then? Since pain is a highly subjective condition, what is needed is a comprehensive, holistic approach to pain management that not only uses drugs but includes forms of complementary therapies such as physical therapy, therapeutic lifestyle modifications, and mindful well-being practices. Pain management must also be tailored to the individual patient; there is no one-size-fits-all approach to managing pain. Guidelines that once recommended opioid drugs as first-line therapy for chronic pain should be reevaluated. And slowly, they are. New treatment guidelines from The CDC for managing chronic pain in the primary care setting suggest that opioid drugs should not be used as first-line treatment. Instead, non-drug and non-opioid therapies should be considered first.[77] When opioid drugs are necessary, it is important to include patients in the decision making process, weigh the risks and benefits, and have realistic treatment goals.

Prescription Stimulants

Another equally concerning, growing trend in prescription drug abuse is the abuse of prescription stimulants. Prescription stimulants are used to treat conditions such as Attention Deficit Hyperactive Disorder (ADHD). Patients with ADHD can suffer from symptoms such as restlessness, impulsive behavior, and the inability to stay focused on tasks. Prescription stimulant medications are used to help people with the disease stay focused to fulfill their daily activities.

Commonly prescribed stimulant drugs include Adderall, Ritalin, Focalin, Vyvanse, and Concerta.

Sadly, prescription stimulants are getting abused by students in high school, colleges, and in adult workspaces, too. They are being illegally sold and abused for the perceived benefits in studying, taking exams, or other project-oriented tasks. According to the CDC, about one in five students have abused a prescription stimulant known as Adderall.[78] Some students even go as far as to fake ADHD symptoms to mislead doctors to write a prescription for them.

But there are serious potential consequences to misusing stimulants. Abusing stimulants or other powerful prescription drugs have serious psychological effects on the brain. Potent prescription stimulants like those described above are classified as Class 2 controlled substances that carry the highest risk of dependency and abuse. Because the brains of young adults are still developing, drug abuse can lead to chemical imbalances that can cause lifelong irreparable damage.

Society puts a lot of pressure on kids to be perfect. The need to get exceptional grades, to be an all-around athlete, to ace the SAT or ACT, to get admitted into the best colleges, or to qualify for a scholarship to help cover the cost of a college education—it can be overwhelming. The pressure to be highly competitive can cause students to turn to drugs to cope with the stress or to get an edge. Parents need to be aware of these dynamics and have ongoing discussions with their children on the topic. It is especially important if the child takes prescription stimulants, pain medication, or other drugs that can be habit-forming. Watch out for these signs of abuse—empty contents of medication capsules, powdery substances or contents of medicine in loose packets, running low on medication after a recent refill, or requesting an early refill multiple times.

But prescription stimulant abuse doesn't only concern the children and young adult populations. Adults are abusing these drugs too. Approximately 25% of adults who go to see a doctor to get a prescription for stimulants like Adderall are faking their symptoms.[79] People who abuse these stimulant drugs do so to get an extra boost of energy and focus. But what they don't realize is that crossing the line from prescription use to abuse can lead to serious consequences that will affect your physical and mental well-being.

The Hard Truth

There are a few hard truths that patients must remember as they work with and take their medications. Understanding these truths is essential to having a healthy and positive health care journey.

- For any health issue, the more involved a patient is with their care and treatment, the better results they are likely to get.
- Patients sometimes do not take their medications as intended or prescribed. Not following your doctor's orders, especially when they involve controlled substances that affect the brain chemistry is unwise. Prescriptions drugs should only be taken exactly as instructed.
- To treat acute pain, pain medications are usually prescribed on an as-needed basis, which means that you should take the medication only when necessary. Always follow the exact instructions given to you by your doctor. Do not double the dose, take more than prescribed, or take it more often than instructed to. For example, if your medication label reads, "Take 1 tablet every 6 hours," do not take another dose after two hours.
- Drug therapy is often marketed as the best solution. Although drugs are a necessary treatment option for many illnesses, medication is not the end-all for many illnesses. Most Americans suffer from chronic health issues that occur over an extended period of time. A comprehensive approach to disease management can be the missing key to the puzzle. Therapeutic lifestyle practices are essential to managing chronic illnesses and should be utilized with medication. Incorporating complementary treatments such as using food as medicine or nutrition therapy, yoga, aqua therapy, sound therapy, meditation, acupuncture, and other

holistic options can help patients cope with the disease by giving them some level of control over their illness.

Teens, Young Adults, and Drug Use

Prescription drug abuse affects teens and young adults. It is important to talk to your older children, especially teens and young adults, about medications and help them learn about the dangers of irresponsible drug use. With the digital age, peer pressure can be a strong contributing factor to young people experimenting with prescription drugs. Prescription drugs used inappropriately can be as dangerous as illegal drugs. Prescription drug abuse by young people is a national problem of epidemic proportions. A third of children aged 12 and over that used drugs for the first time began by abusing a prescription drug.[80]

Even more astonishing is the fact that the majority of people (70%) who abuse prescription drugs obtained these drugs from friends or family; only five percent obtained the drugs through a drug dealer.[81] Among teens 13 to 19 years old, analgesics (pain medications) ranked No. 1, antidepressants ranked No. 2, and sedatives and antipsychotic medications ranked No. 3 among the causes of poisonous exposure, as reported by the Poison Control Centers.[82]

Education is a key factor in preventing drug abuse. We must empower our young adults with information and continue to engage them in open dialogue about medication use and safety. When having such conversations, get the facts so you can dispel the myths. Fact: you can get addicted to a prescription drug. Fact: you can overdose from a prescription drug. Fact: an overdose can lead to serious harm, including death.

Know the facts and dump the myths.

- **Myth:** Prescription drugs are not harmful because they are prescribed by a doctor.
- **Truth:** Prescription drugs can have powerful effects on the body. They can also have side effects. Medication that is abused or not taken as intended can have serious adverse effects on the body.
- **Myth:** Recreational use of prescription drugs is okay. You won't get addicted.
- **Truth:** If you abuse prescription drugs, especially drugs that can be habit-forming, such as narcotics, opioids, sleeping pills, mood, and attention-altering drugs, the risk of chemical dependency and addiction can be high.
- **Myth:** Prescription drug abuse problems only affect certain types of people. It will not affect you.
- **Truth:** Prescription drug abuse can affect anyone. It can affect you, irrespective of race, gender, or socioeconomic status.

Turning it Around

We can no longer turn a blind eye to the problem. No longer can we continue to enable the culture of drug abuse. We have lost too many souls to this crisis. We have lost our mothers, fathers, sons, daughters, uncles, aunts, iconic musicians, and artists in our communities. Opioid abuse is no longer "their" problem; it is "our" problem. We must take ownership of it and act with urgency. For our loved ones, family members, or friends who are caught up in the cycle of abuse, we have to intervene compassionately and get them help. The U.S. Department of Health, Substance Abuse and Mental Health Services Administration at samhsa.gov has treatment resources available to guide you through this process.[83]

Recovery assistance has to come from both private and public partnerships that create and promote accessible, high-quality, and affordable drug recovery treatment programs for all patients. These treatment programs have to address both the immediate and long-term needs of patients. Patients and their families, caretakers, health care providers, and the community at large must understand that there are no shortcuts to be taken because recovery is a lifelong process that requires lifelong treatment.

What can you as the patient do to protect yourself? You should be aware of the risks of the medicines you consume. You should take your medication only as prescribed; do not exceed the dose prescribed by your doctor. Keep your medicines in a secure area. Dispose of any unused medicines promptly. Do not combine medication with alcohol. Do not drive while under the influence of any medication that can alter your state of mind and result in impairment. Be aware that narcotic pain medicines can depress the central nervous system and result in drowsiness. They can also delay your reaction time, affect your concentration and coordination, and cloud your judgment. Patients with chronic opioid use should have Naloxone on hand, which is used to treat and reverse the effects of opioid toxicity. Naloxone can make a difference in life-or-death overdose emergencies. It is available in many pharmacies without a prescription; simply ask the pharmacist for it.

Don't be afraid to seek help if you have a problem with drug abuse. Do not turn a blind eye to a friend or loved one or continue to enable their addiction. The kind and compassionate thing is to reach out and do an intervention. When necessary, consult the services of a mental health provider. An intervention can save a life. If you have a history of an opioid use disorder, be open and honest with your provider. Remember that there are resources to help you and other alternative therapies for pain relief that are available.

In my conversations with patients and caregivers on the front lines, one thing is clear—people are suffering in silence. They are afraid to share or talk about their struggles with their families and even with their health care provider. The fear of being stigmatized is overwhelming and crippling that so many people choose to struggle alone. Moving forward as we tackle this crisis together, I encourage you to not go at this alone. You are not alone in this. The first step in healing and recovery is asking for help. Reach out to a health care provider, get a referral to a mental health counselor and let's do the work to fight this illness together.

Knowledge Checkpoint

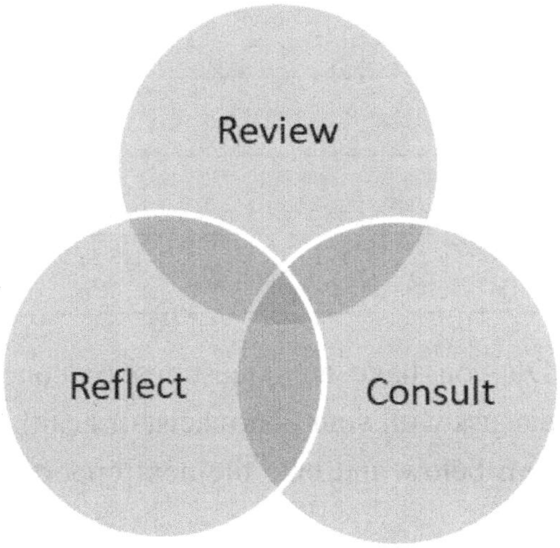

REVIEW: In the preceding three chapters, you have acquired in-depth knowledge about the ways you can save money and time at the pharmacy. Now, you know what to expect when you go to the pharmacy. You reviewed proactive steps to keep you safe and prevent medication errors. You also acquired an in-depth perspective on the drug abuse problem affecting many communities across the country, including yours.

REFLECT: Take a moment to reflect on what you have learned and then answer these questions: Are you currently facing any medication-related issues? The next time you go to the pharmacy, which tips will you use to give you a better experience? What steps can you take proactively to protect you and your loved ones from prescription drug abuse?

CONSULT: Do you have any questions or concerns that you would like to discuss with your pharmacist or health care provider? Write them down below and take the next opportunity to address them.

Chapter 14
Teachable Moments

Pharmacists are asked "Why" a lot. *Why the wait? Why don't you have my medicine? Why isn't my insurance paying for this? Why is my medicine so expensive? Why can't I wait in the drive-through lane until my medicine is ready? Why is that patient taking so long?* Or: *Aren't you just putting a sticker on a bottle? What's taking you so long?*

When such questions arise, I use them as teaching moments to enlighten and educate people about how to make the pharmacy experience as painless and rewarding as possible.

On the job, I love teachable moments. In my view, every encounter I have with a patient is an opportunity to help improve their ability to navigate effectively in the pharmacy world and attend to their medication needs more easily and confidently. Below are some quick tips and light-hearted real life scenarios that have been smile-worthy teachable moments.

Real life Scenarios in the Pharmacy

Here are my Top 10 Tips for a happier pharmacy experience:

Tip 1: If you are dropping off or picking up medication for someone else, you need to be able to identify and validate the patient's information, usually the name, date of birth, phone number, and address of the patient. Having this information will get you in and out of the pharmacy faster.

Patient:	Hi. I am picking up for my grandma.
Pharmacist:	OK. What's her name?
Patient:	Huh? Her name is 'Grandma!
Pharmacist:	Hmmm. OK! What's her birthdate?
Patient:	Oh, I don't know. She's pretty old.

Tip 2: If you can't find your prescription, before you ask the pharmacist about it, ask yourself if someone else in your household might have picked up the medication for you. Always check and verify by simply calling home first. This can make your experience hassle-free.

Patient:	Hi. I want to pick up my medications.
Pharmacist:	Our system shows that your prescriptions were already picked up yesterday.
Patient:	What? No way! But I didn't pick them up. You must have lost them.
Pharmacist:	Sir, that is highly unlikely. Can you call home? Maybe a family member picked them up for you?
Patient:	*(Walking away, calling his wife on his cell phone.)* Oh, you did? (Returns to the pharmacy counter) Oops! My wife picked it up. Sorry.

Tip 3: Stay current with your routine doctor checkups to ensure the continuity of your medications. The pharmacist can't simply give you prescription pills when your doctor has denied the

medication request. Pharmacists do not have licenses to prescribe medications.

Patient: I am picking up my medicine.

Pharmacist: Ma'am, your doctor denied your refill request.

Patient: That can't be true. Why would she do that? I need my medicine now!

Pharmacist: Your doctor says she has not seen you in nearly two years. You have to schedule an appointment with the doctor if you want any refills.

Patient: Oh, I see. Ok. Well, can you just give me some pills because I am out?

Pharmacist: Ma'am, I am unable to do that because your doctor denied your request.

Tip 4: Plan ahead when you are taking vacations or traveling. Don't wait until the last minute to request your medications. Start the refill process at least a few days before you leave. That way, you won't have to worry about running out of your medications when you should be daydreaming about the vacation of a lifetime!

Patient: I am leaving for the airport in 15 minutes, and I need all of my prescriptions filled now. My driver is waiting!

Pharmacist: I will do my best. However, two of the medications you need have no available refills, and another one has to be ordered. I'm not going to be able to dispense them for you in that timeframe.

Tip 5: Before you drop off or pick up medications, and especially if you are new to the pharmacy, be sure that you have all the necessary patient information. This is a standard safety protocol that protects you and your loved ones while the medication is being prepared and dispensed.

> *Patient:* I need to drop off this prescription for my daughter. She's a new patient.
>
> *Pharmacist:* Ok. What is her date of birth?
>
> *Patient:* Hmmm…December 8….No, December 11…2009…No, 2010. Hmmm. Can't you just look it up?

Tip 6: Be kind! Kindness goes a long way in life—and in the pharmacy, too. A way to practice kindness in the pharmacy is to use the pharmacy counters and windows for medication needs primarily so that others that need their medicine or medical care don't have to endure extended wait times.

> *Patient:* Hi. I am here to pick up my medications.
>
> *Pharmacist:* Great! Your total is $16.
>
> *Patient:* Can you run out and grab me a pack of cigarettes with that, too?

Tip 7: Every pharmacy has a standard processing time on medication orders that allows the pharmacist to perform essential safeguards for the medications they dispense. Be patient and factor in the processing time before you head to the pharmacy.

> *Pharmacist:* Thanks for calling. How can I help you?
>
> *Patient:* I just left my doctor's office. Are my medicines ready?

Pharmacist: No, ma'am. Your doctor just sent them over. Give me about 30 minutes for pickup.

Patient: Thirty minutes!! That's too long!

Pharmacist: We just received your prescriptions, and we will need time to review and prepare your medications. I'll do my best to put a rush on it for you.

Patient: That's unacceptable! *(Hangs up.)*

Tip 8: When the doctor gives you a paper prescription, take it to the pharmacy as soon as possible. Even if you do not need it right away, the pharmacist is usually able to hold it on record for you. That way you don't risk losing it. A lost prescription can be a hassle to replace.

Patient: I need a refill of my medicine.

Pharmacist: I am sorry, but you do not have any refills remaining. I can contact your doctor for approval.

Patient: That is impossible. I gave you my prescription last month. It should be on file.

Pharmacist: I am sorry. I am not showing that you dropped off any new prescriptions for this medicine. I can call your doctor to get you more refills.

Patient: Make sure you tell the doctor that you lost my prescription!

(The patient returns to the pharmacy a few hours later.)

Patient: Oh. Hi. Sorry, I found my paper prescription! It was in my wallet all along. When can I pick this up?

Tip 9: It is good practice to know the names of the medications you take. Be able to provide the name of the medication that you need when requesting your refill. This prevents against accidentally requesting the wrong medicine, which can have negative implications to your wallet, health and peace of mind.

Patient:	I need a refill.
Pharmacist:	Which medicine do you need?
Patient:	I don't know exactly, but it's a small, round, white pill.
Pharmacist:	You have several medicines on file that match that description. What is the prescription number on your bottle?
Patient:	I don't have that, either. But I know it's small, round, and white. Can't you just look it up? I'm in a rush.

Tip 10: Pick up your medications as soon as possible after they are ready. Pharmacies have a standby period, keeping prescriptions ready for you for a week or two. If your medications are not picked up during the designated period, they might be returned.

Patient:	I'm here for a pickup.
Pharmacist:	Sorry Sir, I don't have anything ready for you.
Patient:	I requested it over a month ago, and you called me that it was ready.
Pharmacist:	*(Tries to reprocess the order but finds that it has since expired).* Sir, the prescription has expired. You're going to need a new prescription from your doctor.

Patient: But I requested it before it expired. So why isn't it ready?

Pharmacist: It was filled when you requested it, but it was not picked up. The prescription has expired since then, so it's no longer valid. I can send your doctor a request for a renewal and give you an emergency supply.

Patient: No! I need your supervisor now!

Head-scratching, Real-life Questions For a Laugh!

Over the years, I have received some questions that made me chuckle! Here are some for your enjoyment:

- *What aisle is the sugar on?*
- *Is there a sale on ice cream today?*
- *Can I use your cell phone to make a call real quick?*
- *Can you call me a cab?*
- *I am in a rush. Can you just give me one pill right now?*
- *Here's a $20! Can you put a rush on that?*
- *Can you tell my doctor to give me at least eight refills on that?*
- *My car broke down in your drive-through lane; can you come help me move it?*
- *Hypothetically speaking, how do I pass a drug test if I have been naughty?*
- *Can I get an early refill? My dog ate my medicine.*

Chapter 15
Generic vs. Brand-name Drugs

What is a generic drug? A generic drug is biochemically equivalent to a brand-name drug and is known by the name of its active chemical ingredient. It is often a more cost-effective option than the brand-name version. When the drug manufacturer's patent on a drug expires, other drug manufacturers can develop and market generic alternatives as long as they are identical to the brand-name drug and contain the same active ingredients.

Generic medicines are cost-effective therapy alternatives and help keep the cost of your prescriptions down. The Food and Drug Administration (FDA) regulates the process of approving generic drugs and requires that generic drugs be equivalent in quality, potency, purity, and stability as the brand-name drug.[84] As a patient, you can be confident that the generic medicines you receive from a pharmacist meet strict quality standards and are just as good and safe as the brand name.

What is a brand-name drug? When a drug manufacturer holds an exclusive drug patent on a medicine, it is called a brand-name drug. The patent gives the drug manufacturer sole rights to develop and market the drug for up to 20 years.[85] During that time, the drug company has market exclusivity; there is no competition for the drug. Once the patent expires, generic manufacturers can compete to develop and market a generic drug alternative. But they can only do so after thorough testing and approval by the FDA.

At the pharmacy, brand names and generic names of drugs are often used interchangeably—and it can be confusing. Prescription drugs are chemical compounds with one or more active ingredients, and many are available in a generic form. If a generic form of a drug isn't available, it will usually be referred to by its brand name.

For example, if your doctor wrote a prescription for Crestor, but your pill bottle says Rosuvastatin, you need not worry. Rosuvastatin is the chemical name—the generic name—for Crestor. You received the correct medication; it is simply the generic equivalent.

In many states, generic drug substitution is the gold standard. In other words, if a cost-effective generic alternative is available, that's what you'll get unless your doctor or insurance plan formulary prefers otherwise.

If you'd prefer to receive only the brand-name drug for some reason, notify the pharmacist when you submit your prescription. On the other hand, if your doctor prefers that you get the brand-name version, they can write any of the following on the prescription:

- Brand-name only
- Brand-name necessary
- Do not substitute
- Dispense as written

Be prepared. If you or your doctor requests the brand-name version of a medication, it will probably cost you more due to the higher price of the brand name. If you or your doctor *don't* request a brand-name drug, then it's likely you'll automatically receive a generic drug, pursuant to your state's prescribing laws.

Brand Name Drugs and their Generic Equivalents

It's common practice for many different drug manufacturers to manufacturer an active ingredient in its generic form. Here are the brand names and generic names of 75 commonly used prescription drugs:

Brand name	Generic name	Common Uses/Indications
Abilify	Aripiprazole	Mood disorders
Adderall	Amphetamine salt	Attention Deficit Hyperactivity Disorder
Adipex	Phentermine	Weight loss
Aldactone	Spironolactone	High blood pressure
Altace	Ramipril	High blood pressure
Amaryl	Glimepiride	Diabetes
Ambien	Zolpidem	Insomnia
Amoxil	Amoxicillin	Bacterial infection
Atarax	Hydroxyzine	Antihistamine for itching, Anxiety
Ativan	Lorazepam	Anxiety, Insomnia
Augmentin	Amoxicillin with Clavulanate	Bacterial infection
Benicar	Olmesartan	High blood pressure
Ceftin	Cefuroxime	Bacterial infection
Celexa	Citalopram	Antidepressant
CellCept	Mycophenolate	Immunosuppressant
Claritin	Loratadine	Antihistamine for allergies
Coreg	Carvedilol	High blood pressure
Coumadin	Warfarin	Anticoagulant (blood thinner)
Cymbalta	Duloxetine	Antidepressant, Pain
Dilaudid	Hydromorphone	Pain

Duragesic	Fentanyl	Pain
Effexor	Venlafaxine	Antidepressant
Flexeril	Cyclobenzaprine	Muscle relaxant
Flomax	Tamsulosin	Enlarged prostate
Flonase nasal	Fluticasone nasal	Nasal allergies
Fosamax	Alendronate	Osteoporosis
Glucophage	Metformin	Diabetes
Haldol	Haloperidol	Mood disorders
Imitrex	Sumatriptan	Migraine headaches
Keflex	Cephalexin	Bacterial infection
Levaquin	Levofloxacin	Bacterial infection
Lexapro	Escitalopram	Antidepressant
Lipitor	Atorvastatin	High cholesterol
Lovenox	Enoxaparin	Anticoagulant (blood thinner)
Mobic	Meloxicam	Arthritis
Motrin	Ibuprofen	Pain or inflammation
Namenda	Memantine	Alzheimer's disease
Neurontin	Gabapentin	Seizures, Nerve pain
Nexium	Esomeprazole	Stomach acid reflux, Ulcers
Niaspan	Niacin ER	High cholesterol
Nizoral	Ketoconazole	Antifungal
Omnicef	Cefdinir	Bacterial infection
Paxil	Paroxetine	Antidepressant
Pepcid	Famotidine	Stomach acid reducer
Percocet, Endocet	Oxycodone with Acetaminophen	Pain
Phenergan	Promethazine	Nausea and vomiting
Plavix	Clopidogrel	Anticoagulant (blood thinner)

Pravachol	Pravastatin	High cholesterol
Prevacid	Lansoprazole	Stomach acid reflux, Ulcers
Prilosec	Omeprazole	Stomach acid reflux, Ulcers
Pristiq	Desvenlafaxine	Antidepressant
Protonix	Pantoprazole	Stomach acid reflux, Ulcers
Prozac	Fluoxetine	Antidepressant
Requip	Ropinirole	Parkinson's disease
Restoril	Temazepam	Insomnia
Ritalin	Methylphenidate	Attention Deficit Hyperactivity Disorder
Roxicodone	Oxycodone	Pain
Seroquel	Quetiapine	Mood disorders
Soma	Carisoprodol	Muscle relaxant
Tenormin	Atenolol	High blood pressure
Topamax	Topiramate	Seizures, Migraine headaches
Toprol XL	Metoprolol Succinate ER	High blood pressure
Trileptal	Oxcarbazepine	Seizures
Ultram	Tramadol	Pain
Valtrex	Valacyclovir	Antiviral
Ventolin	Albuterol	Asthma
Viagra	Sildenafil	Erectile dysfunction
Vicodin, Lortab, Norco	Hydrocodone with Acetaminophen	Pain
Wellbutrin	Bupropion	Antidepressant
Zanaflex	Tizanidine	Muscle relaxant
Zetia	Ezetimibe	High cholesterol
Zithromax	Azithromycin	Bacterial infection
Zocor	Simvastatin	High cholesterol
Zoloft	Sertraline	Antidepressant

Quick Rx Tip: A brand-name drug will have one unique drug manufacturer since the brand-name patent is exclusive. But a generic drug can have many different manufacturers, which allows for competition and relatively lower costs.

Generic Drugs and their Brand Names

Here are the ten most common generic drugs and their equivalent brand names.[86]

1. Levothyroxine (Synthroid or Levoxyl) - used to treat thyroid disease
2. Hydrocodone/Acetaminophen (Lortab, Norco, Vicodin) - used to treat pain
3. Lisinopril (Zestril) - used to treat high blood pressure
4. Atorvastatin (Lipitor) - used to lower cholesterol
5. Metoprolol (Toprol, Lopressor) - used to treat high blood pressure
6. Amlodipine (Norvasc) - used to treat high blood pressure
7. Metformin (Glucophage) - used to treat diabetes
8. Omeprazole (Prilosec) - used to treat acid reflux
9. Albuterol (Ventolin, Proair, Proventil) - used to treat asthma symptoms
10. Simvastatin (Zocor) - used to lower cholesterol

Test Your Knowledge

Do you know the generic ingredient names of the over-the-counter medications that you use? Test your knowledge and write your answers below.

- Benadryl ____________________
- Claritin ____________________
- Zyrtec ____________________
- Lotrimin ____________________
- Tylenol ____________________
- Advil ____________________
- Aleve ____________________
- Cortisone ____________________
- Lamisil ____________________
- Mucinex ____________________
- Imodium ____________________
- Pepto Bismol ____________________
- Pepcid ____________________
- Allegra ____________________
- Flonase ____________________
- Colace ____________________
- Probiotic ____________________
- Prilosec ____________________
- Gas-X ____________________
- Dulcolax ____________________

(How did you do? See the answers in the Answer Key at the end of this chapter.)

How to Save Money on Brand-name Prescription Drugs

As mentioned, the retail price for a brand-name drug is typically higher than its generic equivalent. As an incentive to use a brand-name drug, some drug manufacturers offer copayment assistance programs that can lower the cost of your brand-name medication. Drug manufacturers market heavily to doctors and routinely provide doctors with drug-specific manufacturer coupons to give to patients upon issuing a prescription. To the patient, drug manufacturer coupons can be thought of as rebates.

Before you can use a drug manufacturer coupon card, the program might require you to complete an eligibility and activation process. The coupon card will come with instructions about how to do that. You can usually activate your coupon card online or by phone. During activation, you might be asked to verify whether or not you have prescription insurance, and you might be asked for other personal information, such as your name, date of birth, address, and contact information. If you have prescription insurance, the type of insurance plan you have might disqualify you from using the drug manufacturer coupon. If your insurance plan is federally funded, as with Medicaid or Medicare, you might be ineligible to use the rebate card.

Once you complete the activation process, your coupon card is activated, and you can present it to the pharmacist with your prescription for additional savings on your brand-name medication.

Drug manufacturer coupon cards don't get processed like the typical coupons you use at the grocery store. You can't just scan, save, and go. It's not that simple! The pharmacist needs to process the coupons electronically, similar to how your prescription is processed with your insurance plan.

Be sure to notify the pharmacist before you pay for the medication that you want to use your coupon card. Like an insurance card, keep your coupon card in a safe place, preferably in your wallet, and present it each time you pick up your prescription. Some coupon cards can only be used once, while others might allow multiple uses. Review the information provided with your coupon card thoroughly, so you are aware of the rules and limitations. Always pay close attention to the expiration date. You might not be able to use it if the card has expired.

Examples of brand-name drugs that offered a copay assistance program at some point during their patent life include Lipitor, Beyaz, Moxeza, Prograf, Metrogel, Solodyn, Benzaclin, Pradaxa, Plavix, Axiron, Ciprodex, Vyvanse, Androgel, Duac, Invokana, Janumet, Belviq, Humira, Crestor, Effient, Eliquis, Harvoni, Humalog, Welchol, Zovirax, Bystolic, Breo, Lotemax, Suboxone, Benicar, Cellcept, Creon, Kaletra, Trokendi, Genvoya, Synthroid, Lialda, Cialis, Viagra, Concerta, Diastat, Diovan, Isentress, Epipen, Ciprodex, Focalin XR, Invega, Januvia, Onfi, Stribild, Uloric, Ozempic, Dupixent, Xarelto, Aimovig.[87]

Test Your Knowledge Answer Key:

Here are the answers to the Test Your Knowledge quiz :

Benadryl: Diphenhydramine
Claritin: Loratadine
Zyrtec: Cetirizine
Lotrimin: Clotrimazole
Tylenol: Acetaminophen
Advil: Ibuprofen
Aleve: Naproxen
Cortisone: Hydrocortisone

Lamisil: Terbinafine
Mucinex: Guaifenesin
Imodium: Loperamide
Pepto-Bismol: Bismuth Salicylate
Pepcid: Famotidine
Allegra: Fexofenadine
Flonase: Fluticasone
Colace: Docusate
Probiotic: Lactobacillus
Prilosec: Omeprazole
Gas-X: Simethicone
Dulcolax: Bisacodyl

Chapter 16
What You Need to Know to Save Money on Health Insurance

Understanding the basics concepts of health insurance will help you save money and time at the pharmacy and help you approach your health care decisions with more confidence and ease.

A health insurance company is a business that purchases health risk. You pay money in the form of a premium to an insurance company, and, in return, they insure your health risk. Purchasing health insurance is a good investment that can shield you from unexpected health care costs and help you secure access to quality health services. Individuals can purchase health insurance through an employer, the government, or on the private market.

Since an insurance company is buying your health risk, any situation that puts you at a greater risk of illness can result in a higher premium. For example, tobacco smokers might pay a surcharge on premiums compared to nonsmokers because smoking carries a higher health risk. You'll likely pay a higher premium, too, if you are insuring a family and not just one individual.

Many patients come to the pharmacy believing that simply because they have insurance coverage, all of the costs associated with their medication are covered. Unfortunately, they are mistaken. Prescription drug insurance works in a similar way as non-medical insurance, such as car insurance.

Think of your health insurance like the auto insurance you pay to cover your car every month. Your auto insurance policy is a contract between you and the insurance company. Your contract is subject to certain benefits, limitations, and deductibles. At the same time, you must maintain your vehicle by performing regular oil changes, brake checks, tire rotation and replacements, engine/transmission services, and so on. Some of the services you have to pay for out-of-pocket, even though they are crucial to the functioning of your vehicle.

Same goes with health insurance. When you buy health or drug benefit insurance, you are agreeing to a contract with your insurance company. You pay the insurance company a premium to buy some of your health or prescription drug liability. The insurance company then assumes some of the risks and pays some of the costs that are related to the medical services or medications you use.

Just like your auto insurance, your health or prescription insurance policy has benefits, limitations, and deductibles, while some services might not be covered under your plan. For example, over-the-counter products, cosmetic products, and non-formulary drugs might not be covered, but like coverage on your car, you still have to do "maintenance" on your health and take care of yourself. Not everything that you do or medicines that you take will be covered by your insurance policy.

So, each time you request a prescription from the pharmacy, your pharmacist files an insurance claim on your behalf. It's like what happens when your car needs repair work, and you need to use your auto insurance to pay for it. Claims in the pharmacy are referred to as prescription drug claims and are subject to the terms and conditions of your insurance policy that you have agreed to, knowingly or unknowingly.

This is why it is essential that you become familiar with the terms of your insurance that you have agreed to. Examine your yearly insurance benefits package carefully when you receive it, so you know what to expect. (Your insurance benefits package is usually sent to you at the beginning of your coverage period. If one is not mailed to you, you might have access to it on your insurance company's website.)

Saving Money on Drug Costs

For those who are not insured, drug prices can be a shocker, and they can present a huge dilemma at the pharmacy counter. An estimated 15% of Americans do not have health insurance.[88] Uninsured patients can often pay full retail price for their medicines—and they can end up being quite costly.

But there's good news. If you do not have prescription drug insurance coverage, there are ways you can save money on your prescription drugs at the pharmacy.

- **Prescription Discount Cards**

  There are drug discount cards available online that you can use to save money at the pharmacy, including Family Wize, GoodRx, Agility Rx, and MedImpact.

  Drug discount cards can save money off of the retail price of a medication, and the savings can be huge. There are many free drug discount programs that you can take advantage of. You can even print a discount card online and keep it in your wallet for easy access. If you have a smart device, you can have it readily available at the pharmacy when you are ready to use it.

  When you plan to use a discount card for a prescription, get it ready before you arrive at the pharmacy. In order to use it, the pharmacist will need the processing information on the card, including the Identification Code, the BIN code, the PCN code, and the Group code.

Only after the pharmacist has processed the information on your discount card can they inform you about the cost of your medicine. You can only use one discount card for each prescription; you can't combine them.

It's helpful to remember that discount cards are *not* equivalent to insurance coverage. The price savings might be minimal, moderate, or astonishing, depending on the medication. Discount drug cards are primarily for those who don't have insurance benefits. Most of the time, insurance benefits offer more savings than discount cards. But a discount card can be very valuable if a drug is not covered by insurance benefits or if you haven't met a large deductible and you have significant out-of-pocket drug costs. If you choose to use a discount drug card instead of your insurance, a big disadvantage is that the money you spend might not get counted towards your deductible. In the event that you have insurance and want to pay down your drug deductible faster, it is best to use your insurance benefits.

- **Pharmacy-specific Discount Programs**

  Many local pharmacies offer programs unique to their specific pharmacy, providing an added benefit for loyal customers. If you get prescriptions filled at a community pharmacy, you should ask your pharmacist if they offer a drug savings program. Enrolling in a drug savings program can help you save money, especially if you use that pharmacy regularly. If your pharmacy does have a discount program, you can ask for a list of covered drugs so you can check if any medications you take qualify for a discount. Since these programs are pharmacy-specific, they might not be transferable or be able to be used at another pharmacy that is not in the same chain network.

For example, when you enroll in a pharmacy savings program at Stella's pharmacy network, you will not be able to use it at Banks pharmacy network because the two pharmacies are not connected or affiliated with each other.

Some pharmacies might offer program discount cards for free, while others might charge a small enrollment fee. Some offer a generic 30-day and 90-day program that provides deeply discounted prices for certain generic medications. Every pharmacy program is different, so be sure to inquire about the specific details with the pharmacist.

- **Patient Assistance Programs**

  These programs, sometimes referred to as "copay assistance programs," are offered by the drug manufacturer for certain brand-name medicines. They help cover some of the cost of select brand-name medications. Sometimes, a drug company might even offer a free trial of a certain quantity of medicine. There are two categories of these patient assistance programs: those for patients that have insurance benefits and those without insurance coverage. The most common programs are typically copayment assistance programs, which help to lower costs for patients who have prescription drug benefits. Depending upon the policies of the program, patients who do not have insurance benefits might not be eligible to use copayment assistance programs due to a coordination of benefits component that is part of the plan. With a coordination of benefits plan, the primary insurance benefit first covers part of the drug cost, and the secondary assistance program supplements the cost.

Patients who have any form of government-funded insurance benefits such as Medicaid, Tricare, or Medicare might not be able to use copayment assistance programs due to federal restrictions. Copay assistance programs vary between brand-name drugs. Some programs are only good for one-time use, while others might be used multiple times with refills. Each program also has a maximum covered value.

Most of the time, information about copay assistance is handed out at the doctor's office when a prescription is issued. When available, some direct-from-the-manufacturer electronic copay coupons are automatically applied and processed by the pharmacy when you get your prescription filled. Always trying to save you money with the resources available, the pharmacist will notify you if they are aware of any programs that might help lower the costs of your medications.

- **Do Your Research**

  When you are taking a brand-name drug, a little research on your part could save you big bucks. Here is how to save money on brand-name drugs:

  Step 1: Find out from the pharmacist if your medicine is classified as a brand-name drug. If so, get the name of the medication and the name of the drug company that manufactures it.

  Step 2: Do an online search of the name of the medication. Look for the official drug website that is referenced by the official drug company. The website will provide information about the medicine and any cost-saving support that is offered by the drug company.

  Step 3: Drug companies often offer ways for you to apply directly and register for available assistance programs online. Or they might direct you to an official hotline where a representative can process your application, answer questions or direct you to additional resources. This process can take 30 to 45 minutes, but it can yield tremendous cost savings. If your application is accepted, you will be issued a physical or electronic card that you can provide to the pharmacist to lower the cost of your medication.

Quick Rx Tip: Although there are different types of discount cards that offer savings on medication costs, discount cards are not equivalent to insurance coverage. For the majority of patients who take medications, especially generic drugs, your insurance benefits will give you the best price on your medication costs.

- **The Truth About Copay Cards**

  Although brand-name copay cards offer patients savings on drug costs, when compared to generic prices, they are not necessarily always a better deal. You should always weigh your options and make an informed choice.

  Here's a personal example. After a visit to my doctor, I was given a prescription for a brand-name drug. Inside the package of information the doctor gave me, there was a free drug sample and a copay assistance card that would reduce my insurance copay down to $25 for a one-month supply. That meant that when I returned to the pharmacy to pick up the brand-name medication, my cost would be $25 each month. Now, $25 per month on one medication might seem to be a great deal. But I wasn't done with my research.

  As consumers, it is sometimes easy to get blinded by coupon marketing. When patients are given a coupon, the automatic urge is to want to use it because it will save us money. But where medications are concerned, a coupon doesn't always offer you the best value. You should weigh your options and make informed decisions with each offer.

Drug manufacturer coupons can often blind patients from knowing the true cost of their medicines. Even if a coupon lowers the cost of your brand-name drug, your insurance still has to pay and cover the cost of the drug. Drug manufacturer copay cards can also push providers and patients towards more expensive brand-name drugs, which directly increases the cost of care.

In my case, my insurance benefits allowed me to get an alternative generic medicine that worked just as well and only cost $12 for a three-month supply. So, I consulted with my doctor, and she agreed to switch to the more cost-effective medication. Every three months, I would pay $12 instead of the $75 coupon price of the brand-name medicine. That's a savings of $300 - $48 = $252 a year on one medication!

Even if you are given a copay card, make it a practice to inquire about the cost difference between a generic product and the brand-name product if one is available. The pharmacist is available to contact your doctor to request a drug change when cost is an issue.

For example, if a generic medicine has a retail cost of $100 and a copay cost of $10, then you'd pay $10, and the insurance company would pay $90. An alternative, brand-name medication might have a retail cost of $350 and a copay of $60. If you use a copay assistance card that lowers the copay to $20, your insurance company still pays $290 ($350 - $60). The manufacturer coupon simply pays $40 of your copay. At first glance, these coupons might seem like a great deal, but, in reality, they can cost you significantly more.

Medication copay cards are becoming increasingly common. Since their inception, their use has increased more than 200%, a troubling trend, because these cards are exclusively for expensive brand-name drugs and primarily target patients with insurance. Retaining patients and solidifying brand-name loyalty is serious business in the pharmaceutical industry. Most of the time, before you can use a manufacturer copay assistance card, you first have to go through an activation process that screens for eligibility. You will likely be asked for your personal information, such as name, date of birth, and address—which the drug company will likely use in direct-to-patient marketing and data-mining campaigns. With all of that personal information they've obtained from patients, drug companies focus on keeping people loyal to the brand, fueling the cycle of continued use of more costly brand-name medicines.

- **Warnings about Copay Cards**

  Copay cards from drug manufacturers can be very confusing to patients. Very often, people only read the front of the card, which mentions some "incredible deal" that they are promoting. For example, the words might state that, with the card, the patient pays only a certain amount for the medication—say, $10. But people often don't pay close attention to the back of the card or the accompanying literature, which has detailed information about the program. If you read the fine print, you will find more eligibility rules and limitations that apply to the program. One of the limitations of copay cards, for example, is the "maximum benefit"— the maximum dollar amount the program will cover. Its dollar value is something you want to pay close attention to. Also, pay close attention to the insurance plans that are not eligible or excluded from using the program.

For example, you might have a copay card that says that you only pay a $25 copay, but the coupon only covers a maximum benefit amount of $50. So, in order for you to be able to get this drug for $25, your insurance copayment must be $75 or less. $75 - $50= $25. Now, let's say that when your pharmacist applies your insurance benefits towards the medication, the copayment is $100. When your pharmacist applies the copay card, your price for this medicine will be $50, not $25. $100 (insurance copay) – $50 (copay card maximum benefit) = $50. Many health care providers with genuinely good intentions often blindly give these coupons to patients without fully understanding the logistics of how they work. As a result, they unintentionally increase the patient's tendency to use costly brand-name drugs, which, in the long run, can significantly increase their cost of care.

Many patients have insurance plans with high deductibles; some can be as high as $5,000. Unfortunately, high deductible plans are increasingly becoming the norm. Patients with high deductible plans have to pay down their deductible before they become eligible for a copayment. That means they pay for a lot more of the cost of their medicines upfront.

For example, a patient received a prescription for a brand-name topical product that had a retail cost of $350. She had a $2,000 deductible on her prescription insurance plan. Because of the deductible, the insurance benefit only covered $40 off the cost of the medicine, which means that although she has insurance coverage, her actual cost responsibility was $310. ($350 - $40 = $310.) She was given a copay card, which, at first glance, implied that she'd only have to pay $30. But the card also had a maximum benefit of $50. When the pharmacist applied the coupon, the final price wasn't even close to $30. Her cost was $260. ($310 - $50 = $260. Her cost, according to her insurance policy, minus the copay card's maximum benefit.

Copay cards will not cover your deductible; they will only cover the maximum benefit amount. There is no way around paying your deductible except for using less expensive drugs to keep the out-of-pocket costs down.

In addition, a lot of drug copay cards cannot be used for patients whose prescriptions drugs are insured under federal or state-funded programs like Medicaid, Tricare, or Medicare because, under these programs, such cards are considered illegal kickbacks. Therefore, it is heartbreaking for me to explain to a patient why he cannot use the copay card his doctor gave him because he has a Medicare Part D prescription plan. He is very upset with me because he was given the card by his doctor. Anything I say to the contrary makes me the bearer of bad news. In situations like this, I believe in full disclosure and try to explain the options that the patient has so they can make the best, informed decision.

When using copay cards, be sure to check the expiration date. A card that has expired cannot be honored. If you receive an expired copay card accidentally, the best thing you can do is to call the program administrator using the customer service phone number located on your card. Speak to a representative and inquire if the program is still active and if the card can be renewed.

The drug company can cancel or change the copay program without any notice. For example, you have been using a copay card with your medicine, and you previously paid $0 because the card fully covered your insurance copay. Now your pharmacist is telling you that your medication costs $25. I understand how frustrating this can be. Unfortunately, the pharmacist does not get an advance warning that your copay card offer is changing. The terms and conditions of these cards are subject to change as determined by the drug company and not the pharmacist. You should always contact the program administrator using the phone number on your coupon card for eligibility concerns or questions.

Quick Rx Tip: You must have a valid prescription before you can use a drug discount card or copay card. I have had interesting encounters with patients who came in to the pharmacy with a drug coupon that they found in the newspaper, wanting me to dispense the medicine to them without a doctor's prescription. This is not possible.

What is Managed Care?

The concept of managed care began out of a need to contain the ballooning cost of health care. Striking the right balance between cost, quality, and affordability continues to be a challenge, but it is a worthy cause. As you navigate your health care needs, be prepared to encounter medical and pharmacy systems that incorporate managed care models such as:

- **Health Maintenance Organizations (HMO):** These health care systems allow patients to seek care within a network of providers. Health care is closely managed using streamlined processes and systems.
- **Preferred Provider Organizations (PPO):** These health care systems allow for patients to seek care from a network of preferred providers that have agreed under contract to a negotiated discount for services. In order for patients to qualify for the negotiated pricing, they must use providers

that are part of the preferred network. Not doing so will result in a higher cost of services.

The cost of care continues to rise, and the goal of cost containment is still as much an issue today as it was a decade ago. Within the health care industry, consolidation, mergers, and resulting monopolies have created a dichotomy that can jeopardize the patient-provider relationship. The choice that patients used to have about which doctor or pharmacy to use is getting narrower and narrower. The autonomy that patients and their providers once had is being challenged.

- Prescription medications are being denied because the insurance wants the doctor to prescribe a different drug.
- Health services and medications are being denied by the insurance company because the plan doesn't consider what the doctor prescribed to be medically necessary.
- Patients have to switch from their established doctors or pharmacists because services are no longer covered under a new insurance plan.
- Medical decisions affecting patient health and well-being are increasingly being taken out of the hands of patients and their health care providers.

Decisions are often being made behind the scenes by for-profit health insurance companies that ultimately align with shareholders instead of what is in the best interest of the patient. Although navigating the complexities of the health care industry can be extremely tasking for both patients and providers, we must continue to use all available resources to promote a higher standard of health care.

Who Pays for Health Care?

In the United States, we have a complex multi-payer system, where different groups share the cost of health care. Over the years, there have been shifts in the cost-sharing dynamic between these stakeholders and, while the cost of health care is shared, it is not shared equally.

Categories of payers that make up the more than 3.6 trillion dollars spent on health care every year:[89]

- Patients/households: 28%
- Federal government: 28%
- Employers: 20%
- State and local government: 17%
- Other private business entities: 7%

Medication Price Quotes

If you have prescription insurance and you need a price quote on your medication, it might be a bit tricky because your pharmacist will need to have your active prescription on record in order to process a prescription insurance claim—even if all you want is a price quote. If you have a hardcopy prescription or you know the specifics of the prescription—drug name, strength, quantity—you can contact your insurance company directly or use your insurance company's online drug formulary database to get an estimated cost of your medication. If you already have a valid prescription on record at the pharmacy, the pharmacist can process it and give you a price quote.

Quick Rx Tip: Even though a pharmacist will ask for your actual prescription to process electronically in order to give you an insurance copayment price quote, you are never obligated to fill the prescription there.

If you do not have prescription insurance and you need to know the price of a drug, the pharmacist can provide you with the retail out-of-pocket price of your medication without having the actual prescription on hand. You will need to provide the pharmacist the specifics of the medication—drug name, strength, and quantity. The pharmacist will still need the actual prescription in order to dispense the medication to you. If a price quote is all you need, you are never obligated to fill the prescription. The prescription can be returned to you or transferred to another pharmacy if you want to shop around for a better price.

Quick Rx Tip: Many pharmacies offer prescription savings programs for patients who do not have insurance, so at the pharmacy counter be sure to ask about any available discounts been offered for patients if you do not have insurance coverage.

Remember, there are also free prescription discount cards that are available online that you can use to lower the cost of your medication, simply provide the pharmacist with the discount codes on the card to save money.

Tips for Managing Insurance, Documents, and More

- Always carry your current insurance card and proper identification with you when going to the pharmacy.
- Like any other form of identification, insurance cards have expiration dates. Make sure that the insurance benefit cards you carry are current. If you mistakenly present an expired card and the prescription claim is processed with it, you might be sent a costly collection chargeback notice.
- If you are a frequent visitor to the pharmacy, it would be helpful to save your insurance company phone number in your phone as soon as you receive your insurance card. The phone number for your insurance member services is located on your insurance card.
- Be sure to read your insurance company's benefits package. It contains valuable information about your coverage and tells you what to expect at the pharmacy.
- If you lose your insurance card, request a replacement card immediately. Your pharmacy insurance card contains processing information that allows the pharmacist to submit a prescription claim.
- In order to bill your insurance company, a pharmacy needs information from your prescription card or pharmacy benefits card, including:
    - Insurance company name
    - Pharmacy (Rx) BIN Number — identifies the health insurance company.
    - Pharmacy (Rx) PCN (Processor Control Number) — identifies and routes the prescription claim to the specific pharmacy's benefits manager.

  - Pharmacy (Rx) ID Number — identifies the patient and is specific to the patient and/or dependents.
  - Pharmacy (Rx) Group — identifies the prescription claim as part of a specific group, such as an employer group.
  - Pharmacy insurance company telephone number in case of processing issues.

- If you have a work-related injury and you are using your employer's workers compensation prescription program, make sure that you receive a copy of your worker's compensation insurance card from your employer, which provides the name of the payor of your medicines, the date of injury, and other important claim information. For worker's compensation-related prescriptions, the insurance claim adjustor may need to approve payment of your medicines. Good recordkeeping and organization on your part can prevent delays in processing and receiving your medicines.
- If you see or hear a drug ad and want to discuss it with your pharmacist, be sure to write down the name of the medication. Without a drug name, "I saw it on TV, " might not be enough information for the pharmacist to help you.
- Use your doctor's visit to ask specific questions about your care and take notes while you are there. The pharmacist will answer your questions, too, but they are not privy to your discussions with your doctor and cannot make assumptions or judgments about your patient-doctor discussions.
- If a loved one is recently deceased, notify the pharmacy they used. The pharmacist will need to deactivate any existing prescription orders.

- If you are a dependent covered under another person's insurance plan, you should have their information readily available, including their name, date of birth, phone number, and address. The *primary insured* is the person whose policy you are covered under, usually a parent or spouse. If you are a covered dependent, the pharmacy may need their information to submit and process a prescription claim. Providing the correct required information could be the difference between your insurance plan accepting or denying your medication.
- Make sure that the information the pharmacy has about you is correct and matches the information your insurance company has, including your name, birth date, phone number, and address. Many insurance companies require the pharmacy to validate this information before they will talk to the pharmacist, and if the information doesn't match, you will experience delays with your prescription order.

Knowledge Checkpoint

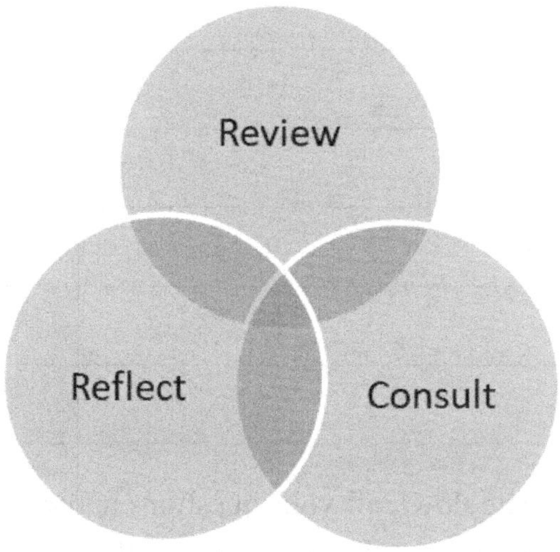

REVIEW: The preceding three chapters highlighted many practical tips that can make your pharmacy experience more pleasant and stress-free. There were real life scenarios that made for teachable moments. You now understand the basic concepts of what a generic or brand-name drug is, as well as the brand and generic names of many commonly used medications. You also reviewed tips on insurance-related concerns and acquired a better understanding of how your prescription insurance works and ways that you can save money on medication costs.

REFLECT: Think about the routine medications you take. Are you able to identify whether they are a generic or brand name drug? How much are you spending every month on your prescription medications? Are you concerned about these costs?

How well do you understand your prescription insurance benefits? Do you have any medication-related insurance concerns?

CONSULT: Write down all your questions and concerns and take the next opportunity to discuss them with your pharmacist or health care provider.

Chapter 17
The Real Power of TLC

Taking your prescribed medications is very important. At the same time, there are many conditions for which medication therapy is not the end-all to achieving healthy living. It is always best to take a holistic, integrated approach and use therapeutic lifestyle changes (TLCs) to maximize and augment your health outcomes.

Though you might be battling chronic health issues, practicing active preventative care through your lifestyle choices is essential if you want to live a happy and healthy life.

Good old TLC. While it's common to think of it as "tender, loving care," "TLC" is the medical acronym for "therapeutic lifestyle changes" that can help you stay healthy. Things that are therapeutic have a healing effect; therapeutic lifestyle changes do just that. In this chapter, you will be introduced to my top 10 recommended TLC's that are guaranteed to improve your health and well-being.

Do not be discouraged if you feel overwhelmed and cannot incorporate all of the recommended changes into your daily routine. Start with one TLC goal and tackle the next. If you fall off the wagon, get back on and keep trying.

To be honest, you have probably already heard of the TLCs that are listed below. There's no top-secret news here. TLCs are not new or proprietary information; your health-care provider will surely remind you of their importance periodically. Even members of your own family who might not use phrases like "TLC" actually encourage you to choose healthier habits and to take better care of your health.

It is our job as medical professionals to assist you in getting healthier, but you must be a responsible, willing participant. Remember, when it comes to our health care system, there are many things that are beyond our control—so focus on the choices you can control. And that means to start with positive therapeutic lifestyle changes.

It's helpful to remember that feeling healthy and being healthy are so much more than a physical thing. Our mental and emotional well-being is also a crucial part of our health. Even with TLCs, it is our mental willingness and fortitude that enable us to begin to try them out and hopefully stick to them. You can build your emotional capital by surrounding yourself with a network of cheerleaders, such as friends, family, and care providers, as you navigate your health journey.

So, begin now. Nurture your mind and body and get on track to a healthier you by putting the following positive therapeutic lifestyle changes into effect.

TLC #1: Quit Smoking Tobacco

If you are a smoker, one of the best things you can do for your body and improve your health is to stop smoking. The statistics on smoking are sobering. Tobacco smoking is linked to half a million deaths per year.[90] An estimated 21% of American adults smoke,[91] and a growing number of children and teens start the habit. Cigarette smoking often leads to tobacco dependency, which is now considered a chronic disease with direct medical costs of $96 billion per year. Smoking increases the risk of stroke, cancer, chronic obstructive pulmonary disease, and asthma and causes other respiratory health issues. Even with these alarming statistics, you might wonder why people continue to smoke. The answer is simple: nicotine.

Nicotine is a highly addictive substance, and cigarettes contain nicotine. When you smoke, nicotine finds its way into your central nervous system (CNS), where it binds to nicotine receptors, resulting in a stimulative effect. The effect gets stronger with continued smoking, and it causes the body to crave more nicotine. That leads to nicotine dependency. When nicotine dependency sets in, attempts to stop smoking can lead to withdrawal symptoms such as shaking, sweating, feelings of anxiety, and changes in mood. As a result, the temptation to continue smoking can feel insurmountable.

Thankfully, there are resources available to help people during the challenges of trying to quit smoking, including:

- Products on the market that contain very small amounts of nicotine and are available in many forms, such as chewing gum, lozenges, and patches. You can use these products to reduce withdrawal symptoms and cravings when you stop smoking. These products are available over-the-counter without a prescription.
- Support groups and hotlines help motivate people to kick the habit and provide positive reinforcement. Free help to stop smoking is available at 1-800-QUIT-NOW. You can also get free help with smoke-free texting programs that allows you to set a quit date and receive daily personalized tips and messages directly to your phone. You can find these resources at www.smokefree.gov.

- Quitting smoking is literally just a click away because there are apps for it! Apps such as quitSTART, also found on www.smokefree.gov, can provide the guidance and support you need. Check out the app store on your digital platforms for innovative apps that can guide you through your journey to quit smoking tobacco.

Here are a few more helpful tips for smoking cessation:

- Instead of taking the kick-the-bucket-down-the-road approach, when you tell yourself you'll stop smoking in the future but never quite get to it, I suggest you try something different. Try this: decide to stop smoking and set a quit date in advance. You already know how to set a date—you do it when you're planning to go out to dinner or the movies, planning to go out with friends, or scheduling a weekend golf trip. Why not add a quit date to the list? You can do it!
- Spread the word. Tell the world! Tell your friends, family, and social network of your decision to quit smoking. There is power in having positive people around you to encourage you. Ask for their support; after all, you will need it. You will be amazed that sharing your journey can motivate you and give you the push you need, and at the same time inspire others to quit, too.
- Focus your thoughts on the positives of life, including the positive things you are gaining from quitting smoking. Mindfulness tools such as meditation, relaxed breathing, focused body relaxation, and mind and body awareness can also help rewire the body's reward system and have been shown to help smokers quit.[92]
- Create a tobacco-free zone by removing tobacco products from your physical environment, such as your car,

workplace, and home. Don't forget that secret stash, too! Out of sight might help keep it out of mind. You want to control the controllable. Granted, you cannot control others if they smoke around you, but you can start with your own personal space.

- The first few weeks after you quit smoking can be challenging, so remember you can use over-the-counter products to decrease withdrawal symptoms. You might have cravings for nicotine, but smoking cessation products can help ease those urges and take the edge off.
- Accept the extra support that is available through support groups, hotlines, and positive reinforcement from your health care provider.
- Keep in mind that your goal is to quit smoking. That means that abstinence is essential. Simply decreasing the number of cigarettes you smoke in a day might not increase your chances of successfully quitting. Talk to other successful ex-smokers for tips and suggestions about how they did it. You are going to need help; do not isolate yourself.
- Rethink vaping, which is often marketed as a safe alternative to smoking cigarettes. Vaping using e-cigarettes or other devices gained popularity in the early 2000s. They use a heating mechanism to turn a solution that usually contains nicotine, flavoring, and other additives into aerosol form. This solution is then inhaled. But more recently, the use of e-cigarettes has been linked to serious respiratory illnesses and has led the Centers for Disease Control and Prevention and the Food and Drug Administration to issue a public warning to consumers on the potential dangers of vaping.[93]

There is encouraging news, though. More and more American's are kicking the habit. Compared to the 1960s, when 42% of adults smoked cigarettes, the number is down to 21%.[94]

The bottom line is this: if you are a smoker, there are a vast number of resources available to help you quit. Many of your fellow Americans have done it, and you can do it, too! In your quit journey, you will find that, like everything else, smoking cessation has turned into a big business, with many drug products, from prescriptions to over-the-counter products, targeting those wanting to quit. In today's world, where health care is commercialized, smokers might find that some smoking cessation interventions push them towards the use of pharmaceutical products they see in targeted prescription drug ads. Remember that you can kick the habit without using prescription medicine. Although we are creatures of habit, and smoking habits can be difficult to break, the idea that individuals cannot quit without taking drugs is false. Most of the clinical research that's been done on smoking cessation is largely funded by drug companies and is primarily focused on drug therapy. The truth is that more people quit without drugs. You just have to find what works for you.

Good luck in your journey! And please inspire others by sharing your journey.

TLC #2: Increase physical activity

Adding physical activity to your daily routine can have a healing effect on your mind and body. The level of physical activity does not have to be strenuous or complex. You can choose activities that you love, such as walking, jogging, dancing, bicycling, yoga, swimming, basketball, soccer, tennis, football, baseball, golfing, or whatever you enjoy. Your options are limitless.

Why physical activity? Physical activity increases your body's metabolism and supports optimal blood circulation throughout your body. It can also help decrease the risk of conditions such as stroke, diabetes, high cholesterol, and depression. Physical activity can also help you maintain a healthy weight and a positive mood. When you actively perform physical activity, the body releases endorphins, natural hormones that are produced by the body that have a positive impact on the body's function. Endorphins have been shown to elevate mood and alleviate pain.

One of the most common questions patients ask me is: What is the best weight-loss product? The truth is there is no magic diet pill that can replace or be a substitute for physical activity. My advice is simply to increase the amount of physical activity you engage in while eating wisely with healthy, nutritional meals. There is no secret, proprietary weight-loss product that can burn all your fat away, although the pharmacy aisles and online marketing are full of products that make those claims. If you incorporate movement and/or exercise into your daily routine and eat wisely, you will feed both your mind and body and likely maintain a healthy weight.

Unfortunately, we are also constantly bombarded with print and online images of what the "perfect" body looks like. So it is important to remember that you do not have to have abs of steel, muscular triceps, and biceps like a fitness instructor, nor do you need a "perfectly" toned body to be considered healthy. Being healthy is not defined by a type of look or a certain number on a scale. After giving birth to four kids, my abs are not made of steel, either! My kids will gladly tell you that mummy's tummy feels like a soft, plushy pillow.

For children and young adults, it is recommended to get at least 60 minutes of daily physical activity at least three times a week.[95] Fun activities can include activities they already enjoy, such as soccer, tennis, ballet, dancing, basketball, volleyball, and baseball.

As for adults, 150 minutes per week of physical activity is recommended.[96] This corresponds to about 20 minutes a day of some form of physical activity. Activities for adults can include walking, tennis, golf, dancing, bicycling, swimming, and gardening. Yet, as simple as that seems, it's easy to find reasons that might prevent us from increasing our physical activity. Many people come home exhausted from work, and all they want to do is eat, take a bath, relax, and go to bed. Also, adults often lose interest in the monotonous routine of working out in the gym and just give up altogether. So, explore the activities you love and that bring you joy, and do it as often as you can! Is there a park or walking trail close by? Simply take a walk. Studies have shown that the simple act of getting outside and interacting with nature has a positive effect on the mind and body, too.

I found that incorporating activities my family enjoys into our daily routine works for my family very well. One of my family's favorite ways to spend family time is to play Frisbee outside. It is a simple, fun, and energizing activity for us that our family can enjoy together. So, take a few minutes of your day, get up, move and have *fun* while you're at it!

TLC #3: Decrease the amount of sodium (salt) in your diet

Ninety percent of our sodium intake comes from salt.[97] Lowering your salt intake can decrease your risk of high blood pressure, heart disease, and stroke. The chemical name for salt is "sodium chloride." Did you know that only 10% of our sodium consumption comes from the salt we actually add to our food during the cooking process or at mealtime?[98] Most of the sodium we consume comes from eating processed and packaged foods. Watch that take-out order, too! Restaurant foods can also be high in sodium. And when you go food shopping, be on high alert for high sodium content and have an awareness of the ingredients in the foods you purchase.

Dietary guidelines recommend limiting sodium intake to less than 2,300mg per day, which is equivalent to one teaspoon of salt per day. For those with chronic health issues such as hypertension, diabetes, and kidney disease, the recommended salt limit is much lower at 1500mg, approximately two-thirds of a teaspoon per day.[99] Be an informed consumer and make informed choices by creating a habit of reading the nutrition labels on foods and selecting low-sodium or no-sodium foods when possible.

When possible, choose fresh fruits and vegetables over canned or processed foods. Foods that are processed often contain added preservatives, which are high in sodium.

As a mother of four, I understand that it is virtually impossible to live without the ease of processed foods. It basically boils down to awareness. The more aware we become of the foods we eat, the ingredients and additives they contain, and the impact they have on our bodies, the easier it gets to make healthier choices.

Quick Rx Tip: Rinsing the contents of canned foods with water and replacing the preservative liquid mixture with water prior to cooking can get rid of some of the added sodium.

TLC #4: Decrease the amount of trans fat foods you consume

Foods made with *trans fats*, also referred to as “trans fatty acids,” and “partially hydrogenated fats,” are artificially made, unsaturated fatty acids and are not healthy to consume. Keep your consumption of them to a minimum. They are chemically engineered by converting and transforming liquid vegetable oils into solid form through a process known as hydrogenation, which adds molecular hydrogen. Trans fatty acids are often used commercially to increase the shelf life of processed and manufactured foods. They are commonly used to make commercially baked or frozen food products such as margarine, donuts, cookies, pies, and pizza.

The Food and Drug Administration (FDA) does not consider it safe for people to consume trans fatty acids.[100] They have been shown to be a double threat to the cardiovascular system. They increase low-density lipoproteins (LDL) in the blood; LDL is known as the “bad cholesterol.” In addition, they lower high-density lipoproteins (HDL) in the blood, which is sometimes known as the “good cholesterol.” HDL can lower your risk of high blood pressure and high cholesterol. The accumulated consumption of trans fatty foods can cause the buildup of cholesterol-filled plaques in the blood vessels, which help to carry blood and nutrients to all of the organs in the body. Key organs, in fact, such as the heart, brain, lungs, kidneys, liver, and pancreas rely on a steady flow of nutrient-rich blood, and compromised blood flow can cause serious organ damage to these key organs. Cholesterol-filled plaques can often become dislodged and cause blockage in blood vessels, which can put you at risk for a heart attack, stroke, or pulmonary embolism.

You might be consuming trans fatty acids without even knowing it. The best way to know if trans fatty acids are present in your foods is by reviewing the nutrition labels of the foods you buy. Keep an eye out for the key ingredient—partially hydrogenated oils. Try to purchase foods that contain either no trans fats at all or that have the least amount of them.

So, what are some alternatives to trans fatty foods? You can get healthy fats from foods such as fish, nuts, and avocados. Naturally, fruits, vegetables, and whole grains do not contain trans fats, so make those your first choice. In addition, instead of cooking with hydrogenated oils that contain trans fats, such as shortening or margarine, use healthier oils such as olive, canola, avocado, or sunflower oils.

TLC #5: Decrease the amount of added sugar in your diet

Added sugar is the sugar that is added to prepared foods during the preparation phase and does not naturally occur in the food. Commercially manufactured foods that contain added sugar include soda, fruit drinks, and baked products such as cookies, cakes, and desserts. How much sugar is good or bad for you? The debate is still ongoing. The U.S. Department of Agriculture suggests limiting added sugar to 10% of daily caloric intake.[101] As a consumer, the most important thing you can do is to be aware of what you are consuming. You can do this by reviewing the nutrition label on the foods you purchase. Recognize that although added sugar makes food taste sweeter, it can be a double threat since it has no added nutritional value, yet it adds calories to your diet. We all have a desire for sweets every now and then, but awareness and moderation are essential. Over time, over-consumption of added sugars can cause obesity and increase one's risk of diabetes.

Managing added sugar consumption is essential to lowering the risk of diabetes as well as complications from diabetes. There are two common types of diabetes. In Type 1 diabetes, insulin production is minimal because the beta cells of the pancreas, which produce insulin, are damaged. Without insulin, sugar that has been consumed cannot be processed; it accumulates and becomes toxic. Patients with Type 1 diabetes have to inject insulin to help digest the sugars they consume. In Type 2 diabetes, damage to the beta cells can lead to inadequate insulin production. Patients with Type 2 diabetes still produce insulin, but not at an optimal level, so they take diabetic medicine to lower their blood sugar to a healthy level.

What can you do to decrease your added sugar consumption? Choose products with less added sugar. Instead of sugary drinks, opt for water for hydration. You can also make your own delicious and healthy juices and drinks fresh by blending your favorite fruits and vegetables into smoothies. Remember that the natural sugar found in fruits and vegetables is always a healthier option than added sugar.

TLC #6: Decrease alcohol consumption

Excessive alcohol use can increase the risk of liver and pancreatic organ damage. It can also have serious side effects when combined with medications. According to the Centers for Disease Control and Prevention (CDC), "excessive alcohol intake" consists of 15 alcoholic drinks or more per week for men and eight alcoholic drinks or more per week for women. Never combine medications with alcohol. Never drive or operate machinery while under the influence of alcohol.

For both over-the-counter and prescription drugs, the side effects and the risk of overdose can increase when they're combined with alcohol. That is because medications and alcohol alike are metabolized through the liver. The liver has a limited capacity of a pint of blood volume that it can metabolize at a time. So, when medicines are combined with alcohol, the liver may not have the capacity to fully metabolize both substances, as a result, high levels of both substances remain in the blood stream, which can cause serious harm to the body.

Many types of drugs, such as those used to treat pain, the common cold, high blood pressure, mood disorders, and diabetes, can have serious side effects when they are consumed with alcohol. Side effects can include drowsiness, dizziness, slowed breathing, impaired motor skills, lapses in memory, seizures, stomach pain, liver damage, vomiting, arrhythmia, changes in blood pressure, fainting, internal bleeding, and ulcers.[102]

It is extremely important that you don't combine alcohol with drugs, especially medications that contain:

- Antihistamines. Antihistamines are found in over-the-counter drugs used for allergies, flu, cough, and cold. Examples: Diphenhydramine, Loratadine, Cetirizine, Chlorpheniramine.
- Benzodiazepines. Benzodiazepines are used to treat conditions like anxiety. Examples: Lorazepam, Diazepam, Clonazepam, Alprazolam.
- Stimulants. Stimulants are used to treat conditions such as attention deficit disorder and hyperactivity disorder. Examples: Methylphenidate, Dextroamphetamine, Lisdexamfetamine, Dexmethylphenidate.
- Pain and anti-inflammatory medications. These medications are used to treat pain and include hydrocodone, oxycodone, butalbital, codeine, methadone,

and acetaminophen. Anti-inflammatory drugs include ibuprofen, naproxen, celecoxib, diclofenac.

- Antidepressants. These medications are used to treat depression. Examples: paroxetine, buspirone, bupropion, citalopram, escitalopram, duloxetine, venlafaxine, amitriptyline, trazodone, fluoxetine, sertraline.
- Anti-diabetic drugs. They are used to treat high blood sugar. Examples: metformin, glyburide, glipizide.
- High blood pressure drugs. They are used to lower blood pressure. Examples: amlodipine, clonidine, losartan, hydrochlorothiazide, benazepril, verapamil, lisinopril, enalapril.
- Cholesterol drugs. Used to treat high cholesterol. Examples: pravastatin, atorvastatin, rosuvastatin, simvastatin.
- Anti-infection drugs. Used to treat infections. Examples: metronidazole, ketoconazole, azithromycin, nitrofurantoin.
- Sleep medicines. Used to treat insomnia. Examples: diphenhydramine, zolpidem, eszopiclone, estazolam, temazepam.

TLC #7: Eat nutrient-rich foods

In today's world, when people swear by a wide variety of diets, and dieting is sometimes the new fashion of the day, remember that the key to healthy eating is to eat for nutrition. To begin, add nutrient-rich foods, such as protein, whole grains, fruits, vegetables, low fat, or fat-free dairy foods. Then, when you eat, use certain safeguards that can be nutritionally beneficial, such as ensuring at least half of your plate contains fruits and vegetables. The benefit you get from eating fruits and vegetables cannot be overstated. They are rich in antioxidants that strengthen the body's immune system, which is your body's line of defense against germs and disease. Eating with an eye for nutrition ensures your body is receiving all of the necessary micronutrients for function and protection. Also, focus on variety in your meal preparation. Food is medicine. While medicine can affect your well-being, the foods you consume can undoubtedly do the same.

The idea that food is medicine is a powerful and empowering concept that is gaining momentum. The point is to teach, encourage, and empower consumers to be aware of what they are feeding their bodies because it has a huge impact on their health and well-being.

Of course, while selecting nutritious foods can have a healing effect on the body, food does not replace your prescribed medications. Medications are used to treat specific conditions and diseases as prescribed by your doctor.

TLC #8: To sleep, perchance to dream

Getting enough sleep is very important. When we sleep, our bodies get to reset and repair. If we spend eight hours sleeping each night, in our entire lifetime, we spend a third of it asleep.

Sleep is integral to our survival; our bodies cannot survive without it. We have a built-in biological clock that regulates our sleep and wake cycle. As we sleep, our bodies go through a complex restoration cycle that results in physiological changes, including the lowering of blood pressure and heart rate, relaxed breathing, and stable core temperature.[103]

The amount of sleep we need varies with our age. The daily recommended amounts of sleep based on age are:

- Newborns (less than three months): 14 to 17 hours

- Infants (4 months to 12 months): 12 to 15 hours
- Toddlers (1 to 2 years): 11 to 14 hours
- Preschoolers (3 to 5 years): 10 to 13 hours
- School-aged children (6 to 13 years): 9 to 11 hours
- Teenagers (14 to 17 years): 8 to 10 hours
- Young adults (18 to 25 years): 7 to 9 hours
- Adults (26 to 64 years): 7 to 9 hours
- Older adults (65 years and older): 7 to 8 hours

Developing good sleeping habits, such as setting a specific bedtime schedule and keeping it, can help us get a better night's sleep. I recommend people first get into *bedtime mode* by taking a warm bath or shower before bed. Set the right ambiance for a night of restful sleep by turning off bright lights and noisy distractions from electronics. Set the bedroom to a comfortable temperature. Besides nighttime rituals, it also helps to incorporate exercise during the day. Also, avoid cigarettes, coffee, caffeine, energy drinks, or a heavy meal close to bedtime.

Insomnia is a common health problem. Gone are the days when there was nothing to watch on television past 9 p.m. Now, with cable TV and on-demand streaming, we have access to 24/7 entertainment that can keep us up late into the night binge-watching our favorite TV shows. Not to mention the array of alerts and notifications our electronic devices send us from our social media accounts and apps.

If you take medicine to help you sleep, you should still practice good sleep hygiene. Only take sleeping medicine when it is necessary. Using it sparingly can decrease the chances of tolerance or dependency to your medication. "Tolerance" occurs when you take a medication regularly and its effects diminish with continued use over time. Eventually, it might begin to feel like the medication is not working. Dependency occurs when you have to take the medicine just to be able to sleep; otherwise, you begin to get withdrawal symptoms. In some cases, patients complain that if they do not take their sleeping medicine, they cannot sleep at all. If you have trouble sleeping, it is important to get to the root cause of your insomnia. Take some time to figure out what that is. If you are like me, a common cause of my insomnia is a snoring spouse. A nice warm lavender bath before bed and soft earplugs usually do the trick.

TLC #9 & #10: Cultivate mental health awareness by developing positive coping skills and using them to manage stress

Learning how to manage and cope with stress effectively is an essential life skill that does not get talked about enough. Stress management is important because the way the body responds to stress can negatively affect our health over time. Our bodies are naturally wired through the flight or fright response mechanism to recognize and respond to stress. Exposure to stress increases the production of natural steroids, such as cortisol and adrenaline, which leads to a cascade of events, including increased blood pressure, heart rate, respiration, muscle tension, blood sugar, and decreased gastrointestinal function. It also slows down digestion, increases gastrointestinal inflammation, can impair memory and concentration, and suppresses the immune system. These cascading stress responses serve as your body's alarm system, a way of alerting you to recognize and avoid danger. Once the stressful event stops, then your body is able to gradually return to normal.

But what if your exposure to stress is a regular occurrence? Or what if you do not know how to manage stress? Then the system is constantly getting activated without any safety controls, and that leads to long-term health consequences.

Stress can affect your physical and mental health, causing symptoms such as muscle tension, headaches, migraines, depression, insomnia, anxiety, overeating, altered mood and cognition, stomach ulcers, and irritable bowel. It can also worsen pre-existing health conditions in those with chronic pain, high blood pressure, diabetes, and autoimmune disorders, making them even harder to manage. Since exposure to stress is inevitable, it is critical that you learn techniques that will help your body repair and reverse the negative effects of the stress response.

The first thing to do to effectively manage stress is to create positive coping mechanisms; the second is to set aside time to practice them regularly. Everyone should have a personal coping plan in place. Coping techniques can be quite simple and can include activities you enjoy doing. For example, you can read a book, practice yoga, go swimming, meditate, try a massage, listen to music, draw, paint, sing, practice counting breaths, write in a journal, volunteer your time to help another person, or simply do something positive that brings you joy. Keep it simple; coping techniques do not have to be complex. The opportunities are endless, and the only criteria are that the activities are positive ones. With continued daily practice, coping techniques can help rewire your body's reward system and, over time, can build your physical and emotional capacity to manage stress.

The unfortunate reality is that, in our quest for healthier living, we often focus mostly on physical health. Sadly, our mental and emotional health does not get prioritized, even though our mental health is just as important as our physical health. From the moment we are born, we are exposed to stress, and it continues through childhood and into adulthood.

Teaching our children about stress management and positive coping skills will help them navigate the stressors of life both in the interim and in the long-term. Teaching stress management skills at an early age can provide children with tools they can continue to use even in adulthood.

There are many techniques that can be used to cope with stress and cultivate mental health awareness. Learning to use one or a combination of them can help counteract the multiplicity of reactions that stress triggers in the body. Practice these skills daily or as often as you can to train your mind and body to stay calm and find peace in the most mundane of things.

Remember that you are not alone; everyone is trying to navigate the many stressors of daily life. The key to success is ultimately how well we use positive, healthy coping mechanisms to deal with our stress. Below are some quick and simple coping techniques that can help ease the stress response in positive and healthy ways:

- **Practice focused relaxation of the body.** When we are stressed, our bodies can react by stiffening up the muscles. Although this is a natural defense mechanism, chronic muscle stiffness can lead to health issues, such as tension headaches and chronic pain. Take five to ten minutes each day to practice relaxing your body from head to toe. Or pick a specific area of the body to focus on, such as the neck, shoulders, or feet. The goal is to teach your body how to relax so that when you do encounter stress, you are able to coach your body to relax at will and reverse stress-induced muscle tension. You can practice focused relaxation in any position—whether you are sitting, lying down, or standing.

Start by breathing slowly and deeply for a few seconds. Then begin to mentally scan your body. Bring your attention to the body as you focus and scan from your feet, legs, abdomen, neck, fingers, hands, chest, shoulders, head, eyes, and so on. As you move your attention through each part of the body, consciously relax the muscles at will. If you sense areas of tension, practice cycles of stretching and relaxing as you continue to breathe slowly and deeply. But keep it simple. This is not intended to be a vigorous or strenuous activity.

- **Practice deep, slow, focused breathing by using the abdominal muscles.** The simple act of breathing comes naturally to us, and we don't think about it much—we just do it. This simple but critical function keeps us alive. Learning how to focus and tap into this natural function can be grounding and invigorating for the mind and body. Focus on each breath as you slowly breathe in through the nose and slowly breathe out through the mouth. Practice for one or two-minute intervals. When we experience a stressful event, the respiratory system can sometimes go into overdrive, and breathing can get rapid and labored. For those with pre-existing respiratory conditions, such as asthma or lung disease, this can be dangerous. Practicing deep and slow breathing can help normalize your respirations during stressful situations by getting needed oxygen into your lungs and tissues.
- **Practice meditation.** By meditating, you can train yourself to be attentive and to be present in the moment. Meditation allows you to focus on tranquility of space, body and mind.

To practice meditation, be in a comfortable environment and position, set a time, such as 15 minutes, and relax your breath and movements and then focus your mind on relaxation. Practice meditation daily for 10 to 15 minutes or as often as you can.

When practicing meditation, you can use what surrounds you—such as things in nature or sights or sounds—to clear and refocus your thoughts. You can also use the power of words, music, or visualization to guide you to a mental state of peaceful calm. Meditation is a good skill to learn and is very helpful when it comes to coping with stress.

Just as we feed the body, we must also feed the mind. Meditation is good nutrition for the mind. By practicing meditation, you teach yourself to nourish your life in the present, which can positively improve your social connections, ease your stress, and get you closer to a happier you.

- **Practice the trifecta of relaxed movement, relaxed breathing, and relaxed mind (meditation)**. The three techniques listed above are commonly used in the practice of yoga, Tai Chi, and Qigong, which are considered complementary medicine because of the verifiable health benefits.[104] The combination of relaxed movements, relaxed breathing, and meditation has been shown to significantly decrease the body's stress response by decreasing blood pressure, heart rate, anxiety, and cortisol production.[105]
- **Practice gratitude daily.** Being grateful is simply the act of recognizing and appreciating the things or the people in our lives. The power of gratitude and the positive effect it has on the body is scientifically proven to increase

happiness, improve health and mitigate stress.[106] So, find ways to be grateful. For example, try keeping a gratitude journal. Take five minutes a day to write down the things in your life that you are grateful for and that bring you joy. The simple act of writing these grateful thoughts down is powerful; by acknowledging and validating their significance, you spark and sustain joy. Often the mere thought of these joyful things can flood your mind with positive emotions that can linger long-term. When you practice gratitude, you develop the skill to stay grounded and mindfully balanced, even in the midst of a stressful environment.

When incorporating gratitude into your daily life, keep it simple. Remember, showing gratitude can be as simple as saying "Thank you" to those around you. With the power of gratitude, you feed your mind good nutrition and unleash the power of positive thinking that can transform your life.

- **Practice kindness daily.** The power of kindness is immeasurable, and performing simple acts of kindness for others is good nutrition for your emotional well-being. You could volunteer your time or services, help someone in need, hold the door for a stranger, give a kind compliment, or help a coworker with a project. The simple acts of kindness we perform every day connect us to our core humanity. Do you ever wonder where that warm, fussy, good feeling you get when you help someone comes from? Being kind has been shown to scientifically increase positive attitude by naturally boosting hormones such as oxytocin, dopamine, and serotonin.[107]

Quick Rx Tip: Your mental health is equally as important to your well-being as your physical health. Take the time and effort to visualize how you will incorporate stress coping practices into your daily life. Take a moment to write down every activity you engage in from the moment you wake up every morning to the time you go to bed. Doing this exercise will give you a working template and help you to schedule your stress management practice opportunities.

As a pharmacist who also practices mind and body wellness, I recommend that you have go-to positive coping plans on standby and consciously and consistently put them into use every day until they become second nature. Doing so can reduce your tendency to reach for unhealthy coping tools, such as alcohol or substance abuse, that have a negative impact on your well-being. Plan to implement healthy wellness practices daily to help you succeed. How do you achieve this? Start by using personal notes, a journal, or a planner to set your personalized coping goals. Program reminders on your personal devices to help you stay on track. You can also share your journey, seek out support, and learn more about whatever mind and body wellness techniques spark your interest. Ultimately, having a proactive mental health wellness plan will equip you with tools to manage stress and transform your outlook on life.

Set specific goals for yourself to help you succeed. Here are some examples:

- I will start my day every morning doing five minutes of focused body stretches and relaxation.

- Before I go to bed every night, I will write down five things that bring me joy.
- On my drive to work every day, I will meditate for five minutes.
- The next time I get angry or frustrated, I will focus on my breathing for five minutes.
- When I feel overwhelmed at work, I will take a mental power break and meditate for five minutes.
- Every day, I will make a commitment to do one random act of kindness for a stranger.
- Once a week, I will volunteer my time or resources to help someone.

The beauty of setting up a healthy mindfulness lifestyle to cope with stress is that it does not have to cost you anything; it is free. The opportunities are endless, and the reward is truly intrinsic. They are simple techniques that both young and old can master and learn to boost their capacity to handle stress and to live a healthier, happier, and more well-balanced life.

Safe Use of Dietary Supplements

Dietary supplements are health products that contain vitamins, minerals, herbs, botanicals, amino acids, or other dietary ingredients that are regulated under a different set of guidelines than prescription and other over-the-counter drugs.[108, 109]

The use of dietary supplements in the United States is big business, with tens of thousands of dietary supplements available to consumers. Annual sales of dietary supplements top over $100 billion, and sales continue to grow as patients focus on proactive preventative care.[110] As patients are willing to spend top dollar on dietary supplements, they are often deluged with false and misleading claims about supplements, and separating fact from fiction can get difficult. One cannot deny the power of drug advertising, and companies that make dietary supplements spend a lot of money on direct-to-consumer advertising through all types of media. A trip down the supplement aisle at your local pharmacy can leave you bewildered and amazed at the endless variety being offered. Products come in different forms—tablets, capsules, powders, gummies, liquid gels, chewables, liquid solutions, quick-dissolve tablets, etc.—and there are many companies that make the same products.

Although dietary supplements are generally beneficial and safe to use, you should still be cautious when choosing them. Currently, there is only limited regulatory control over the manufacturing and distribution of these products. Just because a dietary supplement is referred to as "natural," "vitamins," or "herbs," it does not imply or guarantee the safety or purity of the product. Do your research and consult with a health care provider, such as a pharmacist, before use. The pharmacist is usually just a few steps away from the supplement aisle; it would be worth your while to consult with one.

Before you purchase any dietary supplements, be sure to review its list of active and inactive ingredients on the package and carefully review any warning labels for potential health risks. Still, even doing your due diligence does not always guarantee that you are 100% certain of the exact content of the supplements you are consuming. Independent testing of some dietary supplements on the market has shown that these products sometimes don't contain the ingredients mentioned on the label, and sometimes they contain unlisted ingredients.[111]

Currently, the FDA does not review the efficacy or safety of dietary supplements. With the passage of the Dietary Supplement Health and Education Act (DSHEA) in 1994, the manufacturers of dietary supplements do not have to prove that their products are safe or effective.[112, 113] There is limited oversight over this industry, and manufacturers are not required to register their products with the FDA or get approval before producing or selling dietary supplements.[114] The FDA can only take action against an unsafe product after it reaches the market. Since the FDA does not regulate them, manufacturers of dietary supplements are responsible for establishing their own manufacturing guidelines, and that means that the identity, purity, quality, composition, and strength of their products can be questionable.[115] This regulatory loophole can result in potentially unsafe dietary supplements getting marketed to consumers.

Also, keep in mind that special populations such as the elderly, patients with kidney or liver disease, children, pregnant women, and patients with complex chronic health conditions are at a higher risk of experiencing adverse effects and should take extra caution when selecting a dietary supplement.

This is not to say that dietary supplements don't have their place in patient care. They absolutely do. They offer a convenient way to obtain nutrients outside of consuming them naturally in food. However, although they are classified as nutritional supplements, they are often commercially manufactured with added ingredients like gluten, sugar, sodium, artificial coloring, gelatin, yeast and preservatives.

Quick Rx Tip: If you choose to use a dietary supplement, be sure to do your research prior to purchase, buy only from reputable sources, read the ingredient label carefully, and only use products that lists both active and inactive ingredients. Select products that contain a higher percentage of active ingredients versus inactive ingredients. For example, if a supplement lists the total active ingredient as 2% but it contains 98% inactive ingredients, of which 90% is sugar--this may not be a healthy choice.

Some of the commonly used dietary supplements include:

- Aloe Vera: used as a topical skin remedy for burns and wounds.
- Biotin: used for hair loss and brittle nails.
- Black Cohosh: used to relieve symptoms of menopause or premenstrual syndrome.
- Calcium: used to maintain strong bones, muscle function, and teeth.
- Echinacea: used to stimulate the immune system.
- Folic acid: used to facilitate a healthy pregnancy.
- Ginger: used to relieve nausea.
- Glucosamine: used to help with pain relief from osteoarthritis.
- Iron: used in the production of red blood cells that carry oxygen throughout the body.
- Lactobacillus probiotic: used to aid in digestion and prevent diarrhea.
- Magnesium: used to regulate muscle and nerve function.
- Melatonin: used to help regulate sleep.

- Vitamin A: used to stimulate the immune system and support good vision.
- Vitamin C: used to stimulate the immune system.
- Vitamin B6: used to aid in metabolism.
- Vitamin D: used to maintain strong bones and aid in the absorption of calcium.
- Vitamin E: used to stimulate the immune system.
- Zinc: used to stimulate the immune system and help with wound healing.
- Saw Palmetto: used to relieve urinary symptoms associated with enlarged prostate.
- Omega-3 fatty acids: used to support cell membranes in the eyes, brain, heart, and lungs.[116]

Chapter 18
Medication Safety

Protecting Children from Accidental Poisoning

Accidental ingestion of medication by children is dangerous and even fatal. Curiosity can often get the best of little children, especially toddlers, who may think that a medication is candy and unintentionally take something that is not intended for them. So it is extremely important not to leave medications within reach of young children.

Sadly, accidental ingestions of medicines by children are on the rise; they account for the majority of emergency room visits and admissions of children.[117] Accidental medication poisoning can occur with prescriptions and nonprescription drugs, including dietary vitamins. Making matters worse, our country is facing an opioid epidemic, and many American homes keep highly potent and dangerous medications that can be fatal to a child.

A very common cause of child accidental poisoning is access to Grandma or Grandpa's medications, accounting for about 20% of unintended intoxication in children.[118] Since elderly patients often have difficulty opening standard pill bottles, they often use easy-to-open medication organizers. But when pill organizers are left unattended or within reach, children can easily get into them.

Infants, toddlers, and young children cannot distinguish between safe and unsafe medications. It is, therefore, our responsibility as caretakers to protect them from an unintentional mishap. Anyone in the presence of young children must ensure medicines are kept away, out of sight, or locked up.

Do not underestimate the intelligence of your toddler or young child. They are smart and can use a stool or chair to reach into a cabinet. If you have children in the house, it's a good idea to use child safety locks to secure your medicine cabinets. Be aware that tamper-resistant pill containers can give a false sense of security. Even though you use tamper resistance containers, a child might still be able to open the bottle.

Finally, medicines aren't the only things that can be dangerous! Be careful about where you store cosmetics products, too! They, too, can be hazardous to children if ingested.

Quick Rx Tip: An important note for parents: anyone watching your children, such as grandparents, caretakers, and babysitters, should be instructed not to leave medicines out around them. When your child is visiting with friends or family outside the home, make sure the home is child-proof with no medications left on countertops, in coat pockets or in bags within easy reach.

Whether you are a parent or a caretaker, take the following steps to prevent your child from accidental exposure to medications:

- Don't place medicines in arm's reach of young children. Medicines should be locked up or stored away where they are not accessible to young ones. When children are around, do not leave medicines on the table or countertop. Also, be sure to remove any pill bottles from the pockets in your clothing. If you keep medicines in your purse or handbag, be sure to secure them away, too.

- Don't place purses or handbags containing medicine on the floor.
- Don't refer to medicines as "candy" in front of children.
- When giving a child their medicine, always give the exact dose written on the label. Do not give more than the prescribed dose. More is not better!
- When possible, use child-resistant caps on medicine bottles. But remember that child resistance caps do not mean it is fully child-proof.
- If your child asks you what you are doing when you're taking your medicine, make it a teachable moment. Talk to them at a level that is appropriate for their age. Teach them that it is never okay to take a medication that belongs to someone else.
- When you give a young child their medicine, let them know that only an adult is allowed to give them their medicine. Young children should not self-administer medication. And older children still need adult supervision.
- Don't keep medications you don't need. Dispose of medications that have expired or are no longer needed.
- Don't place discarded medications in the trash inside your home. When disposing of medications at home, use coffee beans or cat litter to mask the odor, place them in a tightly sealed bag or container, and dispose of them in the trash receptacle outside the home. If your pharmacy is a registered drug disposal site, you might be able to dispose of your used medications at the pharmacy. Check with your pharmacist about returning unused medications.

- In case of unintentional exposure to medications, call The National Poison Control hotline at 1-800-222-1222. It is a 24-hour free hotline that is staffed by poison-control specialists.
- When young children visit others outside the home, be sure to remind caretakers, relatives, and friends to child-proof their home.

Topical drug products—products that are placed directly on the skin for fast absorption—can also be the cause of accidental poisoning, so be sure to take similar precautions with them as well. Topical formulations can come in patches, creams, ointments, gels, and solutions. If you are wearing a medication topically, such as a patch, if possible, keep the area covered so that it's not visible to a child. Children can get exposed to the topical drugs if they access an unsecured medication stash or by pulling them off the skin of an unsuspecting adult, and they might place the medication in their mouth.[119]

Here are two cases of actual at-home accidental poisoning of children:

- An infant found a Fentanyl patch—a powerful narcotic opioid used to treat severe pain—and put it in his mouth. The child was found unconscious. Fortunately, the child survived after treatment in the hospital.
- A toddler found a Fentanyl patch and applied it to his body. Unfortunately, his parent found him dead.[120]

In a report by the Poison Control Center, the primary cause of adult exposure to poisonous substances was due to analgesics pain medications.[121] For children, exposure to analgesic pain medications ranked third. The report also showed that more than

90% of the accidental poisoning cases occurred due to exposure at home, and almost half of the cases occurred in young children younger than six years old. The top ten causes of poisonous exposure in young children less than six years of age are:[122]

1. Cosmetics and personal care products
2. Household cleaning products
3. Analgesics (pain medications)
4. Toys
5. Topical/externally applied medications
6. Antihistamines in cough and cold medications
7. Vitamins
8. Pesticides
9. Dietary supplements and herbs
10. Plants

Remember that any kind of exposure to drugs can cause serious harm to a child and can result in a traumatic health scare. But it also can be avoided. That is why prevention is key. Parents, grandparents, guardians, and caretakers must stay vigilant about preventing children from gaining access to potentially dangerous medications in the home.

Medication Disposal

My philosophy about medication disposal is this: If you don't need it, toss it. If you don't use it, toss it. If it's expired, toss it. If you're done with it, toss it.

When you do dispose of medications, do so safely. People often get into the habit of stockpiling unused medications that are either expired or that they're not taking any longer. That's not a good idea. I often get calls from patients asking me if they can use medications that have expired months or even years previously. Sometimes they ask if they can give them to a family member or friend. The answer? Absolutely *not*! Get in the habit of routinely going through your medicine stash, for example, every three months, and safely discard all expired, old, and unused medications. Do not share or give others your unused prescription medications.

Prescription drugs are to be used only by the intended patient. Giving your prescription drugs to someone else can result in harmful effects.

Billions of prescription pills get dispensed to patients every year, and many of them go unused. In one year alone, over four billion pills were dispensed to patients at the retail level.[123] Imagine how many unused medications are sitting in household cabinets across the country—the number is hard to fathom. In one year alone, a record total of 456 tons of unused pills were collected across the country in DEA-approved drug take-back events.

You can safely dispose of medications in several ways. First, before disposing of the prescription bottles, be sure to remove any personal information on the bottle itself.

- Always follow the disposal instructions on your medicine handout.
- Take the medication to a pharmacy that is an authorized and registered drug disposal site. Check with your pharmacist about the approved sites in your local area. You can also find a registered medication disposal site by going to the official DEA website at DEA.gov.
- Purchase a medication disposal mail-in pouch if one is available over-the-counter at the pharmacy.

- Take your prescription to a community prescription disposal take-back event. These community outreach events are organized by the DEA on a local level and are usually advertised in the community. The DEA website, DEA.gov, is also a good resource for information about dates and sites of prescription take-back initiatives.
- You can safely do it yourself at home. Mix the medication with cat litter or coffee beans to mask the odor. Place that in a tightly sealed bag or container and dispose of it in the trash receptacle outside the home. Avoid placing in the trash bin inside the home due to the risk of access by children or pets.

Chapter 19
Electronic Rx, Automatic Refills, and Prescription Adherence

Electronic prescriptions

Electronic prescriptions, also known as "eRx," are quickly becoming a common, convenient, and efficient way for doctors to send patient prescriptions directly to a pharmacist. It is easy and convenient for you, the patient, too, because you don't have to deal with handling a physical prescription that could get lost or damaged. It definitely saves time because you bypass the entire "drop off" process altogether. For pharmacies, the advantages are that they decrease the "paper shuffle," and since electronic prescriptions are computerized, they are more legible. As electronic prescribing is becoming more prevalent, it is helpful to keep in mind a few things to ensure a seamless pharmacy experience:

- There is often a lag time between when the provider sends the eRx to the time it reaches the pharmacy. Some go to the pharmacy immediately after their doctor visit, expecting their medicines to be ready to go. Often, the eRx order has not even arrived yet.
- It is helpful to you and the pharmacy if you verify the status of your eRx order before you go to the pharmacy to pick it up. Electronic prescriptions go through the same review

process as any other prescriptions, so be sure to allow sufficient time for the pharmacy to carefully and accurately fill them.

- Sometimes eRx's are unintentionally sent to the wrong pharmacy by the prescribing provider. It's a good idea to verify with your prescriber the phone number and address of the pharmacy they are sending the eRx to prevent confusion.

Automatic Medication Refill

Many pharmacies offer automatic medication refills to make it easier for patients to adhere to their maintenance medications. With this service, the pharmacist can refill your medicines for you automatically without you having to request them on your own. Once you opt in to the program, your medicine automatically refills about the same time every one to three months. The service is ideal for patients that are on long-term maintenance schedules for chronic illnesses that are dispensed every one, two, or three months. These might include medicines for:

- Contraception
- Blood pressure
- Diabetes
- Cholesterol
- Osteoporosis
- Rheumatoid Arthritis
- Thyroid disease
- Asthma or pulmonary disease
- Alzheimer's and Parkinson's disease
- Gastrointestinal disease

Automatic medication refills can be convenient, but the practice does have its limitations. It works great in theory, but there are many variables and technical hiccups that are prone to occur. It is not suited for use with acute medications that you only need every so often. Medications such as antibiotics or pain medications following a surgical procedure are used for acute conditions. These are not reoccurring, so they are not appropriate for automatic refill.

Automatic refills are made possible by a computer-generated program that can have technical flaws, so it can make mistakes that lead to medication errors, too. In fact, the technical glitches are too common to ignore. If you choose to opt in to an automatic medication service, use it as a secondary tool in your medication organization routine; do not use it passively or rely solely on it. Elderly patients and those taking multiple chronic medications need to be especially careful when using this service.

When picking up an automatic refill prescription, for example, never assume that the medicine you wanted is the one that you are getting. Prior to checkout, always ask what you are receiving before you pay and leave the pharmacy to ensure you are getting exactly what you expected.

Most pharmacists spend a significant amount of time every day fixing automatic refill order issues. Some of the common concerns that arise include:

- Patients arrive at the pharmacy expecting to pick up an order that is not there because the automatic refill system failed to reprocess it.
- Sometimes the system fails to recognize that the same order is ready, so it automatically fills duplicate prescriptions for the same medication.

- The system might automatically refill a medicine that is to be used for an acute—not chronic—condition, and the patient only intended to use it once. For example, a patient received an order of promethazine and tramadol. Promethazine is a nausea medication, and tramadol is used for pain. After five days, the system automatically refilled the promethazine order because it had a refill attached, even though the patient hadn't requested it. The patient called the pharmacy, asking why the order was refilled when she didn't need it. The pharmacy responded by cancelling the automatic refill. When a medication that you do not need gets automatically refilled, notify the pharmacist so it can be manually taken off of automatic refill.
- Some automatic refill systems automatically notify a prescriber to change a 30-day order of medication to a 90-day supply. This practice of converting 30-day prescriptions to a larger quantity might be beneficial for certain patient situations, but with some kinds of drugs, such as psychiatric medications, the practice can be extremely inappropriate and potentially harmful. The American Psychiatric Association has expressed concern regarding the practice of dispensing high quantities of psychiatric medications to patients when a small supply was originally authorized because access to high quantities of psychiatric medications can lead to an increased risk of overdose or suicide.[124]
- Doctor's offices are being bombarded with automatic computer-generated refill requests from pharmacies. Some doctors complain that such requests are often not authorized by the patient, they are inappropriate, and they increase workload, leaving them with piles of such requests

to sort through. As a result, patients can inadvertently continue medications that are only intended to be used for the short term.[125]

- The automatic refill date of a drug is usually based on the last time it was dispensed to the patient. A patient might not be able to identify a specific date to get the medication refilled in the future or synchronize all of their medications so that they are refilled at the exact same time. Trying to synchronize all the drugs that a patient is taking to refill automatically at the same time is a noble but often difficult task due to insurance quantity limitations, drug shortages, ordering delays, prior authorizations, and more.
- Some insurance plans contractually don't allow a pharmacist to automatically refill a medicine.
- Automatic refill systems might accidentally refill a medicine that has changed or that you don't need any longer. For example, your prescription for labetalol for high blood pressure is on automatic refill. Your doctor recently changed your dose to one tablet three times a day, but the system refilled your old prescription for one tablet two times a day. In some instances, the automatic refill system might even auto-refill *both* prescriptions.

Quick Rx Tip: If you use an automatic refill service for your medications, stay vigilant and be sure to always check to know the drugs you are picking up before you pay and leave the pharmacy each time.

Notify the pharmacist immediately if your doctor discontinues a drug or if there has been a change in therapy or dose. The pharmacist needs to update your prescription record and deactivate the medicines you no longer take to prevent them from being inadvertently refilled in the future. Also be sure to notify the pharmacist if you decide to discontinue the automatic refill service or if you have moved and no longer need the service.

Medications can keep cycling through the automatic refill process on repeat and never get picked up by the patient. It ends up being a waste of time for the pharmacist and tie up needed inventory. Be sure to contact your pharmacist if you no longer need or want a prescription that is being filled for you by automatic refill.

Adherence

Taking your medicines as prescribed plays an important role in your getting well, while non-adherence can be costly to your health and well-being. For a lot of people, staying compliant with a medication regimen can be a struggle. If taking your medications correctly is a challenge, you are not alone. Statistics show that 20 to 30% of prescriptions that doctor's issue never gets filled. Moreover, about half of patients taking medications for chronic illness do not take their medications correctly [126]

Some of the most common reasons people find it hard to adhere to prescribed regimens include:

- The cost is high or unaffordable
- Side effects are unpleasant or perceived to be unpleasant
- Preexisting stigma and misinformation regarding medicine use
- The medical issue involves complex disease management, requiring multiple medications
- There are physical or cognitive challenges
- Language barriers
- Forgetfulness

Never abruptly discontinue your medication without discussing it with your provider. Talk to your doctor or pharmacist about your concerns. No matter how challenging your situation might be, there are always other options available. Have open and candid ongoing discussions with your health care provider about any actual or perceived barriers to your treatment plan, beginning when you first start a new medication and throughout the course of therapy.

The importance of adhering to your medication treatment plan cannot be overstated. Chronic health conditions such as high blood pressure, heart disease, and diabetes are silent killers. They might not give you warning signs or symptoms that let you know a serious problem is erupting.

Prescription noncompliance can put your health at risk; it increases the risk of morbidity and mortality, resulting in up to 150,000 deaths per year.[127] When things come up that make it difficult for you to follow your medication treatment regimen, notify your health care provider as soon as possible. If there are cost issues, have your pharmacist call your doctor to see if there is a less expensive alternative. If you get side effects from your medication, remember that side effects can often become less burdensome or resolve completely once your body adjusts to the medicine. If medication side effects persist, then talk to your doctor to explore your other options.

You can find creative ways to ease or avoid minor side effects. For example, if a medicine causes nausea or has a bad taste, you can take it with food to reduce the uncomfortable effects. If a medicine causes drowsiness, take it as an evening or bedtime dose. If you have fears, anxiety, or any concerns about a medication or need more information about a drug, simply stop by the pharmacy and speak with the pharmacist for advice. If you are taking a lot of medications and find the regimen too complex or confusing, talk to your doctor about using combination pills that might decrease your pill burden. Or have the pharmacist come up with a better pill schedule that will work for you. If you have language or physical challenges that negatively affect your adherence to your medicine, ask for special accommodations to address your specific needs.

Quick Rx Tip: Many pharmacies offer an array of tools and services that can help with medication adherence. You can simply choose the tools that work for you. For example, automatic refills, adherence and reminder alerts, and digital tools that notify you when it is time to fill your maintenance prescriptions can be tremendously helpful.

Knowledge Checkpoint

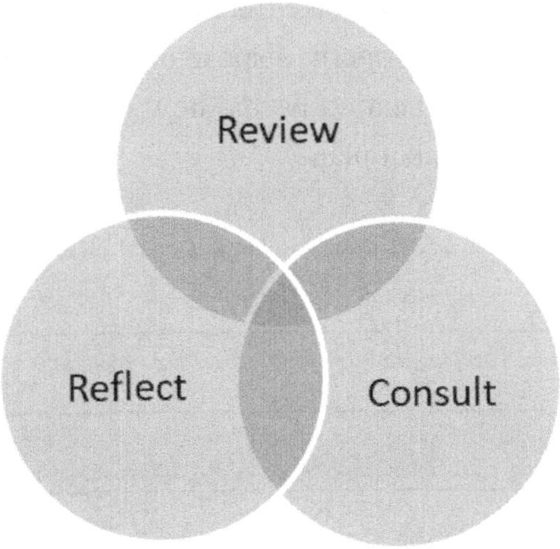

REVIEW: In the preceding chapters, you reviewed therapeutic lifestyle changes (TLC) that have positive effects on your health and tips to improve your physical and mental health. You reviewed best practices for safely choosing an over-the-counter dietary supplement. You also learned about the importance of keeping medications secured and the steps you need to take to safely dispose of unused drugs. Finally, you reviewed the best practices for using electronic prescriptions and learned about automatic refill services and some solutions for improving medication adherence.

REFLECT: Take a moment to answer these important questions: What are your TLC goals? Do you have a positive coping plan to manage stress? Which stress management techniques do you plan to incorporate in your daily routine? Are there other techniques that pique your interest for further exploration? Are all the medications in your home properly secured? If not, then take the necessary precautions to secure them. What types of safety precautions will you take to protect the young children in your household from medication accidents? If you have any expired medications in your cabinet, take the time to go through your entire medication supply and properly dispose of all expired drugs. Think about your unique medication needs, how compliant are you with your medication treatment plan?

CONSULT: On your next visit with your trusted pharmacist or health care provider find out if their facility can dispose of unused medications. Also, discuss any concerns that you have about your medications or health needs. Together, find solutions to address them.

A Glossary to Help You Master the Pharmacy Experience

For the best possible experience with your pharmacy, I strongly encourage you to learn and understand the language of your pharmacist. Whether you get prescriptions from them very often, occasionally, or just once in a while, knowing these words and concepts will help save you a lot of frustration. After all, you don't want to be the one at the pharmacy counter that's holding up the checkout lane, arguing with the pharmacist about why your pill bottle says "Simvastatin" when your doctor told you he was giving you Zocor—with everyone around you looking at you like you're from another planet! (I'll explain the mystery later in this chapter. If you want to jump there now, read about generic drugs below.) Here are the most important terms for you to understand as you work with your pharmacist to have the best possible experience.

30-Day Supply

This implies that you have received a one-month supply of your medicine. Doctors often authorize prescriptions in monthly intervals for maintenance prescriptions that are taken every day. For example, if you received a prescription for 90 tablets of Hydralazine 25mg, and you are to take one tablet three times a day, it is a 30-day supply. (90÷3=30)

90-Day Supply

This is a three-month supply of medicine. For convenience, you might want to request a larger quantity of medicines you take routinely and daily, and the maximum will be 90 days.

Many insurance companies, especially prescription Medicare plans, allow patients to get a three-month supply of medications. Check with your insurance company for terms and availability.

Annual Deductible

The annual deductible is the total amount you must pay each calendar year for covered health services or medications before your full insurance plan benefits, such as copayments and coinsurance, go into effect. For example, if you have a $2,000 annual deductible, you will have to pay that down before your full insurance benefits begin. The annual deductible is a very important detail of your plan that you should carefully consider when you choose your plan. Annual deductibles vary widely, from as low as $50 to as high as $7500 or more. As health care costs grow, the insurance market is shifting more of the cost burden to patients. Patient annual deductibles are on the rise, and high deductible plans are now the norm. Over the past decade, I personally have gone from no-deductible plans to having a deductible of $5,000. Even with employer-sponsored insurance plans, high-deductible plans are now a take-it-or-leave-it deal, where "leave it" means you don't have insurance coverage at all.

Brand-name Drugs

These are drugs that have no generic legal substitute. A brand name drug is made by one manufacturer which holds an exclusive drug patent.

Coinsurance

Coinsurance is a formula for cost-sharing, where you—the insured patient—and the "insurer"—the insurance company—

share a predetermined percentage of the cost of services or drugs.

For example, an 80/20 coinsurance formula has the insurance company paying 80% of the cost and you, the insured, paying 20% of the cost. For example, if the retail price of your medicine is $350, your insurance will cover $280 (80%), and you will pay $70 (20%).

Copayment

The prescription copayment, also known as a "copay," is a predetermined rate or price you pay for covered services. It is your share of the cost for services rendered. Services include doctor visits, prescriptions, emergency room visits, laboratory testing, diagnostic services, and other medical procedures. Your copayment is determined by your insurance plan based on the specific plan you have. Some prescription copayments are structured using a tiered formulary system. The following is a hypothetical example—the copay structure for a tiered-based system will vary based on the specific plan formulary:

- Tier 1 medication (generic drug): $0 to $25
- Tier 2 medication (preferred brand drug): $26 to $45
- Tier 3 medication (non-preferred brand drug): $46 to $100
- Tier 4 specialty medication: $100 or more

Are you concerned about your copay? You are not alone. More and more of the cost of drugs is passed down to the patient. If you do find yourself in price shock when you pick up your medicine, instead of arguing with the pharmacist, take a moment to call your insurance company. As I've mentioned, all questions about copayment pricing should be directed to your insurance company because the pharmacist does not determine your copayment.

Once your prescription order has been submitted and processed, your pharmacist *can* tell you:

- Your copayment amount (your share of the cost)
- The actual, full cost, or *retail price* of your medicine
- How much of the actual cost was covered by your insurance policy
- Whether it is classified as a brand or generic medicine
- If your insurance company has informed your pharmacist, your pharmacist can also tell you whether a deductible was factored into the cost of your medication

Your health insurance policy is a contract between you and your insurance company, so your pharmacy does not know why your copayment or deductible is a certain amount. In fact, you need to direct all of your "Why" questions to your insurance company. When you call your insurance about a drug, be sure to have ready the following information to get the fastest and most accurate feedback. At your request, the pharmacy can provide you with the information:

- Your insurance member ID number
- The drug name and strength
- National Drug Code (NDC): A unique sequence of numbers that identifies the drug
- The quantity and days of supply of medicine

Days of Supply

This is the duration of medication therapy—the number of days you are to use a medicine. For example, if you pick up 20 tablets of Doxycycline, an antibiotic, and your doctor wants you to take one tablet two times a day, you will be on the medication for 10 days. Therefore, the days of supply would be 10 days.

Drug Compounding

This is the process of mixing specific ingredients, per your doctor's prescription, to make a medicine for you. Examples include diaper rash ointment, mouth wash, hormone therapy, and topical creams. Not all pharmacies have compounding services. You might need to go to a specialty compounding pharmacy for complex compounding services.

Drug Formulary

As described earlier, a drug formulary is an approved list of drugs that are covered under the insurance plan.

Drug Not Covered

A "drug not covered" rejection is a claim denial from your insurance company, stating that the prescribed medicine is not covered by your insurance policy. When this happens, you have a critical decision to make. You can choose to pay out-of-pocket for your medication, or you can have the pharmacist contact your doctor to switch to a different drug that is covered by your insurance. You could also pursue an appeal with the insurance company through a prior authorization process.

Drug Not in Stock

The phrase means that the pharmacy does not have the medication you are requesting in stock. But if the product is available from the manufacturer, the pharmacist can usually order it for you.

Emergency Supply

An emergency supply might be allowed in a few situations when you run out of refills on routine medications such as blood pressure, heart, or seizure medications when your doctor cannot be reached. Your pharmacist might be able to give you a limited three- to five-day emergency supply, so long as you have a current refill history on record at the pharmacy. This does not apply to medications that are controlled substances.

Generic Drugs

These drugs are available in a generic form that is bioequivalent and essentially similar. Generic drugs are a lower-cost alternative compared to brand-name drugs. For example, the generic name for Zocor is “Simvastatin.” The drug is used to lower cholesterol. (Remember the scenario I described earlier when the patient’s prescription was for Zocor, and what he received was a generic Simvastatin? Here’s why that happened.) The two are one and the same. It is routine to use the name of a drug’s active ingredient—its generic name—when referencing a brand-name drug.

Insurance Appeal

You can pursue an appeal on a denied medication claim from your insurance, such as when a prior authorization request was denied. If you want to pursue this route, be sure to contact your insurance company and get the information and forms needed to do so. Typically, you'll have to submit a letter stating why you believe the insurance company should approve your appeal or claim. During an insurance appeal, it is helpful if your doctor writes a letter of support for your case. Having personally gone through the process myself, I understand how aggravating and disheartening it can be for patients. It is extremely hard not to get emotional when your health is on the line. My advice is to be persistent, get clarity from your insurance company on what is needed of you, complete your paperwork on time, and know that the rest is out of your hands.

Medication History

This is your prescription history at a pharmacy. It contains details such as the names and dosages of your medications, the prescribing doctor, the dates received, and the cost. Medication histories can be useful at your doctor's office or when you need to do your end-of-year tax filing.

Non-Preferred Drugs

A non-preferred drug is a drug that your insurance might not cover or will charge a higher copayment for because it is not listed on the insurance drug formulary. It is usually more expensive for you to purchase than a preferred drug.

Original Date

The *original date* is the date that a prescription is issued or written by your doctor, and it is used to determine when a prescription expires. A prescription for a non-controlled medication is valid for one year from the original date, while a controlled medication is valid for six months. Some states might have different rules. Refer to your pharmacist.

Over-the-Counter Drugs (OTC)

OTC drugs don't require a prescription from a doctor; you can purchase them over the counter. OTC drugs are prepackaged with directions for use on the bottle.

Pharmacy Benefit Management (PBM)

Have you ever wondered why you have two different insurance cards for your medical versus your pharmacy benefit? Say, for example, you chose United Health Care for your health benefit, but when your insurance cards arrived, you got two cards. One is a medical card from United Health Care, and the other is a pharmacy card from Express Scripts. You wonder, "What is Express Scripts, and why am I getting a card from them?"

A PBM is simply the company that is contracted with your health insurance company to administer and streamline the pharmacy benefit portion of your insurance plan. Pharmacy prescription claims are usually billed instantly at the point of service. When a prescription is processed, your pharmacist needs to know right away whether your medicine is covered and how much your payment should be. Also, if the prescription is not covered, the pharmacist needs to know the reason for denial, what alternatives are covered, and if an appeal is applicable. The PBM serves as a portal or middleman between the insurance company and your pharmacy.

Preferred Drugs and Drug Formularies

There are literally thousands of prescription drugs available to treat a plethora of health conditions, and not all of them are covered by your insurance plan. That's when a drug formulary comes into play. A *drug formulary* is a comprehensive list of all the drugs that are covered under your insurance plan. When a drug is classified as a *preferred drug*, for example, it simply means that it is on the insurance company's drug formulary: it is covered by your insurance plan.

Insurance companies use the services of Pharmacy Benefit Management (PBM) companies to manage drug formulary decisions. Based on cost alone, one would assume that drugs that are less expensive compared to others in the same therapeutic class would be on the drug formulary. Unfortunately, this is not the case due to complex non-transparent contracts, rebates, and deals between key stakeholders such as drug manufacturers, insurance companies, and PBMs. I have had too many head-scratching moments when a relatively cost-effective drug has been denied by the insurance company while a drug that is significantly more expensive is accepted. If you want to know what medications are on your insurance drug formulary list, a good place to find out is your insurance company's website.

Prescriptions and Refills

Your prescription allows the pharmacist to dispense medication to you in predetermined intervals, as instructed by your doctor. Your medicine might or might not have refills, depending on the duration of therapy determined by your doctor. A prescription refill simply means your doctor has given approval for you to continue the medication. For example, if you have one refill listed on your medication, you can refill your medication order just one time after you have gone through the original supply.

Prescription Drugs

Also referred to as "Rx" drugs, prescription drugs require a doctor's prescription to be purchased from the pharmacy.

Prescription Transfer

This is the process of transferring a prescription between pharmacies. For example, if you have had your prescription filled at Pharmacy A, but now you want to get it filled at Pharmacy X, it would be a prescription transfer. To make this happen, you'll need to notify the pharmacy where you want to start picking up the medicine and give them the authorization to transfer your prescription. They will then initiate a transfer request on your behalf and will notify the pharmacy that has the prescription of your transfer request. Once the request is received, your prescription information will be transferred verbally or electronically.

If both pharmacies are part of the same business chain, the transfer can be done electronically for eligible non-controlled medications. Prescription records are treated the same way as medical records; they are secure and confidential. Proper protocols must be followed with no shortcuts, so keep that in mind when you are transferring prescriptions. It is often easier and faster to transfer prescriptions between the same pharmacy chain because they share the same computer systems.

Prior Authorization

A *prior authorization*, or *coverage determination*, is a process by which your doctor can petition your insurance company to cover a drug that it doesn't usually cover. Your doctor will complete and submit a prior authorization form that includes details of your existing health condition, other therapies that failed, and proof or reason for medical need. The insurance company will then review the request and either approve or deny it. Unfortunately, the prior authorization process can cause delays in getting your medication. Sadly, at this point, you are at the mercy of the insurance company. If you encounter a need for prior authorization on a medication, notify your doctor immediately and ask your insurance company for an expedited resolution.

Keep in mind that, during the prior authorization process, the pharmacist may not have much leverage to do anything to expedite your cause. They simply serve as the liaison between the doctor and the insurance company.

Refills Not Covered

This phrase often suggests that your insurance might not cover your requested refill and implies that your insurance company might want you to get your medication from another source, such as a mail-order service or a specific pharmacy. When this occurs, contact your insurance company promptly to find out what you need to do to set it up, opt out, or inquire about other available options.

Refill "Too Soon" or "Too Early"

Both of these phrases tell you that the prescription is not due for a refill yet based on the last time the medicine was filled. For example, if you picked up 90 tablets of your cholesterol medicine Pravastatin 40mg on April 15, and you are taking one tablet daily, your next refill date will be on or around July 15—in three months or 90 days. If you try to refill it again on April 30, your insurance will deny the order because it is not yet time for another refill. Similarly, if the doctor sends an order for a medicine that is not due to be filled yet, the insurance can also deny the order.

Knowledge is power. Stay informed

and be an active partner in your care.

Best wishes in your health and wellness journey.

About the Author

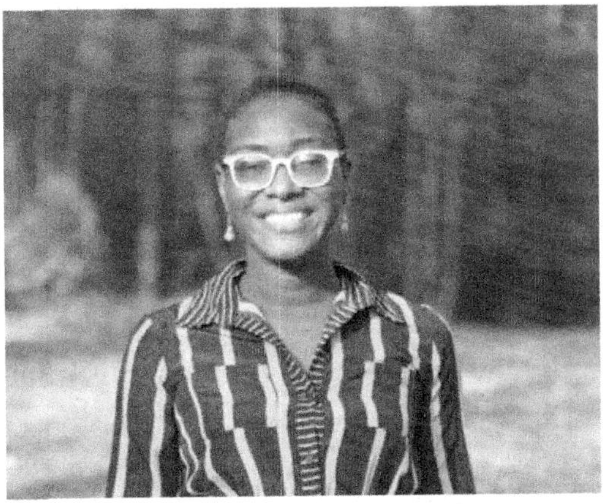

Dr. Ibiyemi Odetola Brown, Pharm.D is a pharmacist, wellness coach and joy scientist. She received a Doctor of Pharmacy degree from the University of Texas in Austin and Mindfulness-Based training from Yale University. She specializes in mind and body wellness, and has spent 20 years in front-line community health care, helping patients navigate their medication and health care needs. She is a passionate patient advocate who loves helping others use the science of joyful wellbeing to live happier and healthier lives.

Dr. Brown is the CEO and founder of Six Joys, a health, wellness and lifestyle brand focused on mental health education. The mission of Six Joys is just that—simply joy! It is to teach and inspire people to live, love and share joy and to cultivate a life of wholesome wellbeing. She lives in Atlanta, Georgia with her husband and children.

Stay connected with Dr. Brown on **sixjoys.com** and on social media using **@joyscientist**

Book Review:

If you found this book helpful,
leave a book review on the Author's page

https://www.amazon.com/author/ibiyemibrown

Books By The Same Author:

The Joy Scientist Joy Journal

ENDNOTES

---

[1] Office of Prescription Drug Promotion, U.S. Food and Drug Administration, Division of Drug Marketing, Advertising and Communications. FDA.gov.

[2] Center for Medicare and Medicaid Services. "CMS Office of the Actuary releases 2017 to 2026 Projections of National Health Expenditures." February 14, 2018.

[3] Ibid.

[4] Ibid.

[5] Ibid.

[6] Ibid.

[7] Pharmacists: A Profession People Trust." *Drug Topics*. January 8, 2019. https://www.drugtopics.com/article/pharmacists-profession-people-trust.

[8] Patricia M Barnes, Barbara Bloom, and Richard L. Nahin. "Complementary and Alternative Medicine Use Among Adults and Children: United States, 2007." National Center for Health Statistics, Centers for Disease Control and Prevention. 2008.

[9] Ibid.

[10] NPR. "Insured, But Indebted: Couple Works 5 Jobs to Pay Off Medical Bills." December 26, 2018. https://www.npr.org/sections/health-shots/2018/12/26/678749817/insured-but-indebted-couple-works-5-jobs-to-pay-off-medical-bills.

[11] Institute for Safe Medication Practices. "What's in a Generic Name? Clues About the Drug's Use and Possible Adverse Effects." March 9, 2017. https://www.ismp.org/resources/whats-generic-name-clues-about-drugs-use-and-possible-adverse-effects.

[12] Ibid.

[13] D. E. Farrell, B. Jensen, N. Kochner, et al. "Accounting for the Cost of U.S. Health care: A New Look at Why Americans Spend More." Washington, DC: McKinsey Global Institute, 2008.

[14] American Association of Poison Control Centers. "2016 Annual Report of the American Association of Poison Control Centers' National Poison Data System (NPDS): 34th Annual Report. Clin Toxicol (Phila)." 2017.

[15] Mark Cuter, Elizabeth Greenberg, Ying Jin, and Christine Paulsen. "The Health Literacy of America's Adults: Results from the 2003 National Assessment of Adult Literacy (NCES 2006–483)." Washington, DC: U.S. Department of Education, National Center for Education Statistics, 2006.

[16] Cuter, M., Greenberg, E., Jin, Y., and Paulsen, C. (2006). The Health Literacy of America's Adults: Results From the 2003 National Assessment of Adult Literacy (NCES 2006–483). U.S. Department of Education. Washington, DC: National Center for Education Statistics.

[17] Drug Enforcement Administration news release. http://www.dea.gov.

[18] Kaiser Health News. "Study: Malpractice Costs $55.6 Billion Annually, Most In Defensive Medicine." June 11, 2020. https://khn.org/morning-breakout/malpractice-7/.

[19] U.S. Department of Health and Human Services. "Treating Tobacco Use and Dependence: 2008 Update." Tobacco Use and Dependence Guideline Panel, Rockville, MD. May 2008.

[20] World Health Organization. "Medicines: Rational Use of Medicines." 2010, http://www.who.int/mediacentre/factsheets/fs338/en/.

[21] Stephen W. Schondelmeyer and Leigh Purvis. *Rx PriceWatch Reports*. Washington, DC: AARP Public Policy Institute: 2019.

[22] Ibid.

[23] *JAMA 310*(1.8):1942-1963. (2013)

[24] Ibid.

[25] Victoria Knight, "American Medical Students Less Likely to Choose to Become Primary Care Doctors." Kaiser Health News. July 3, 2019.

[26] Wikipedia. January 6, 2016.

[27] Diana Farrell, Eric Jensen, Bob Kocher, Nick Lovegrove, Fareed Melhem, Lenny Mendonca, and Beth Parish. "Accounting for the Cost of U.S Health Care: A New Look at Why Americans Spend More." McKinsey Global Institute, 2008.

[28] Aaron S. Kesselheim, Michelle M. Mello, and David M. Studdert. "Strategies and Practices in Off-label Marketing of Pharmaceuticals: A Retrospective Analysis of Whistleblower Complaints." *PLoS Med 8*(4): e1.00043. ssdoi:101371./journal.pmed.1.000431.

[29] Ibid.

[30] Ibid.

[31] The Economist. July 7-13, 2012, 61.

[32] Blake Ellis and Melanie Hicken. "Cashing in on Dementia Patients, Drug Maker to Pay $1.1.6 Million in Fraud Settlement." CNN. September 26, 2019.

[33] Don Peterson. "Origins of an Epidemic: Purdue Pharma Knew its Opioids Were Widely Abused." *New York Times*, May 29, 2018. NYTimes.com.

[34] Charles Ornstein. "We've Been Tracking Pharma Payments for Nearly a Decade. We Just Made a Big Breakthrough." Propublica. December 20, 2019.

[35] Ibid.

[36] Childbirth connection.org.

[37] *Harvard Political Review*. "How Insulin Became Unaffordable." Harvardpolitics.com.

[38] U.S. State Dept. State.gov.

[39] Rayhan A. Tariq, Rishik Vashisht, and Yevgenia Scherbak. "Medication Errors." Updated June 15, 2020. In: StatPearls [Internet]. Available from: https://www.ncbi.nlm.nih.gov/books/NBK519065.

[40] U.S. Food and Drug Administration. "Drug Shortages." https://www.accessdata.fda.gov/scripts/drugshortages/.

[41] Patient Safety Network, Agency for Healthcare Research and Quality. "Medication Errors and Adverse Drug Events." January 2019. https://psnet.ahrq.gov/primer/medication-errors-and-adverse-drug-events.

[42] Ellen Gabler. "How Chaos at Chain Pharmacies is Putting Patients at Risk. *New York Times*. January 31, 2020.

[43] Drug Information handbook. 14th edition.

[44] Agency for Healthcare Research and Quality. April 2011. http://www.ahrq.gov/consumer/safemeds/yourmeds.htm.

[45] U.S. Food and Drug Administration. http://www.fda.gov/Drugs/DrugSafety/DrugShortages/ucm050796.htm. October 14, 2011.

[46] U.S. Drug Enforcement Agency. https://www.dea.gov/drug-information.

[47] American Hospital Association. *Fast Facts on U.S. Hospitals, 2018*. Aha.org.

[48] Sarah Fader. "What is Dopamine and How Does It Affect the Brain and the Body?" Betterhelp.com. May 9, 2019.

[49] Ibid.

[50] Office of National Drug Control Policy. "Epidemic: Responding to America's Prescription Drug Abuse Crisis." Washington, DC. 2011.

[51] Centers for Disease Control and Prevention. November 2011. http://www.cdc.gov/VitalSigns/pdf/201.1.-1.1.-vitalsigns.pdf.

[52] Ibid.

[53] Ibid.

[54] Ibid.

[55] CNN. "Fentanyl is the deadliest drug in America." CNN.com. Dec 12, 2018.

[56] Centers for Disease Control and Prevention. November 2011. http://www.cdc.gov/VitalSigns/pdf/201.1.-1.1.-vitalsigns.pdf.

[57] (2018) *Pain Manag Nurse 1*(2): 125-129.

[58] Ibid.

[59] Ibid.

[60] *The Washington Post*. "Generic Drug Companies Played a Central Role in the Crisis." July 30, 2019.

[61] Ibid.

[62] Ibid.

[63] *The Washington Post*. "76 Billion Opioid Pills: Newly Released Federal Data Unmasks the Epidemic." July 16, 2019.

[64] Ibid.

[65] Henry J Kaiser Foundation. "Opioid Overdose Death." August 8, 2019. https://www.kff.org/state-category/health-status/opioids/.

[66] Ibid.

[67] McKinsey Global Institute, 2008.

[68] Ibid.

[69] Henry J. Kaiser Foundation. "Opioid Overdose Death." August 8, 2019. https://www.kff.org/state-category/health-status/opioids.

[70] Politico. "Drug Overdoses and Suicides Fuel Drop in U.S Life Expectancy." https://www.politico.com/story/201.8/1.1./29/suicide-overdose-life-expectancy-1.025922.

[71] Ibid.

[72] *The Washington Post.* "Drilling into the DEA Pain Pills Database." July 21, 2019. https://www.washingtonpost.com/graphics/201.9/investigations/dea-pain-pill-database/?utm_term=.21.93f8a72ddc#download-resources.

[73] CBS News. "Opioid Shipments Ballooned as an Addiction Crisis Grew, Data Shows." July 17, 2019.

[74] Office of Public Affairs, U.S. Dept. of Justice. Press Release Number 20-1136. October 21, 2020. https://www.justice.gov/opa/pr/justice-department-announces-global-resolution-criminal-and-civil-investigations-opioid.

[75] Ibid.

[76] The United States Department of Justice. Office of Public Affairs. October 21, 2020. Press Release Number 20-1136. https://www.justice.gov/opa/pr/justice-department-announces-global-resolution-criminal-and-civil-investigations-opioid.

[77] Centers for Disease Control and Prevention. "Guideline for prescribing opioids for chronic pain." August 10, 2019.

[78] ABC news. "Adderall Alters Brain, Claims a Young Life." November 8, 2010. Abcnews.go.com.

[79] Ibid.

[80] International Narcotic Control Board. "Narcotic Drugs: Estimated World Requirements for 2011. Statistics for 2009." United Nations. http://www.incb.org/pdf/technical-reports/narcotic-drugs/201.0/NAR_201.0_EFS_Part4.pdf.

[81] Ibid.

[82] 2016 Annual Report of the American Association of Poison Control Centers' National 2016 Annual Report of the American Association of Poison Control Centers' National Poison Data System (NPDS): 34th Annual Report. Clin Toxicol (Phila). 2017.

[83] SAMHSA. https://www.samhsa.gov/find-treatment August 10, 2019.

[84] Manasseh HR, Speedier MK. (2007) "Pharmacists, Pharmaceuticals, and Policy Issues Shaping the Work Force in Pharmacy." *American Journal of Health-System Pharmacy 64*(1.2): e30-e48.

[85] Ibid.

[86] *Drug Store News*. 2016 Report. p. 12.

[87] Medicare.gov.

[88] U.S. Dept. of Health and Human Services. "Treating Tobacco Use and Dependence: 2008 Update." Tobacco Use and Dependence Guideline Panel. Rockville, MD. May 2008.

[89] California Healthcare Foundation. *2020 Edition--Heath Care Costs 101*. May 26, 2020. https://www.chcf.org/publication/2020-edition-health-care-costs-101/.

[90] Office of the Assistant Secretary for Health, U.S. Dept. of Health and Human Services." Ending the Tobacco Epidemic: A Tobacco Control Strategic Action Plan for the U.S. Department of Health and Human Services." Washington, DC: 2010.

[91] Ibid.

[92] Judson A. Brewer, Sarah Mallik, Theresa A. Babuscio, et. al. "Mindfulness Training for Smoking Cessation: Results from a Randomized Control Trial." *Drug Alcohol Depend 119*(1.-2): 72-80.

[93] U.S. Food and Drug Administration. "Lung Illnesses Associated with Use of Vaping Products." September 27, 2019. https://www.fda.gov/news-events/public-health-focus/lung-illnesses-associated-use-vaping-products.

[94] Centers for Disease Control and Prevention. "Smoking Cessation." http://www.cdc.gov/Features/SmokingCessation.

[95] Centers for Disease Control and Prevention. Physical Activity Fact Sheet for Adults.

[96] Ibid.

[97] Centers for Disease Control and Prevention. "Sodium Fact Sheet." http://www.cdc.gov/salt/pdfs/Sodium_Fact_Sheet.pdf.

[98] Ibid.

[99] Centers for Disease Control and Prevention. "Physical Activity Fact Sheet For Children and Adolescents."

[100] American Heart Association. January 19, 2019. Heart.org.

[101] U.S. Dept. of Health and Human Services and U.S. Department of Agriculture. *2015 – 2020 Dietary Guidelines for Americans*. 8th edition. 2015. Available at https://health.gov/our-work/food-and-nutrition/201.5-2020-dietary-guidelines/.

[102] National Institute on Alcohol Abuse and Alcoholism. “Harmful Interactions Mixing Alcohol with Medicines.” Pubs.niaaa.nih.gov. Publication no 1.3-5329. 2014.

[103] Francesco Cappuccio, Michelle A Miller, and Steven W. Lockley, *Sleep, Health and Society: From Aetiology to Public Health*. New York: Oxford University Press, 2010.

[104] *Int J Yoga 4*(2):49-54.

[105] Ibid.

[106] M. Chowdhury. “The Neuroscience of Gratitude and How It Affects Anxiety and Grief.” *Positive Psychology*.

[107] “The Science of Kindness.” Cedars Sinai. February 13, 2019. https://www.cedars-sinai.org/blog/science-of-kindness.html.

[108] American Society of Health-System Pharmacists. “ASHP Statement on the Use of Dietary Supplements.” *Am J Health-Syst Pharm 61*(1) 707-711.

[109] U.S. Food and Drug Administration. “Dietary Supplements.” March 15, 2005. www.cfsan.fda.gov/~dms/supplmnt.html.

[110] Reuters. “Dietary Supplements Market Size, Growth, Statistics, Trends, Segmentation, Demand, Product-Type, Attractiveness, Top Companies Analysis, Business Opportunities and Forecast 2019-2024.” May 14, 2019. https://www.reuters.com/brandfeatures/venture-capital/article?id=1.08942.

[111] Office of the Attorney General of New York. “Attorney General Schniederman Announces Major Nationwide Agreement with Herbal Supplement Maker.” January 25, 2018. ag.ny.gov.

[112] American Society of Health-System Pharmacists. “ASHP Statement on the Use of Dietary Supplements.” *Am J Health-Syst Pharm 61*:1707-1711.

[113] U.S. Food and Drug Administration. “Dietary Supplements.” www.cfsan.fda.gov/~dms/supplmnt.html. March 1.5, 2005.

[114] Ibid.

[115] Fontanarosa PB, Rennie D, DeAngelis CD. “The Need for Regulation of Dietary Supplements: Lessons from Ehedra.” *JAMA 289*:1568-1570.

[116] Office of Dietary Supplements, National Institutes of Health. May 23, 2020. https://ods.od.nih.gov/factsheets/list-all/#.

[117] McPhee RB, Carpaccio TR. "'Hang up your pocketbook'—An Easy Intervention for the Granny Syndrome: Grandparents as a Risk Factor in Unintentional Pediatric Exposures to Pharmaceuticals." *JAOA 106*(7): 405-411. Accessed at http://www.jaoa.org/cgi/content/full/1.06/7/405.

[118] "Vital Signs: Overdoses of Prescription Opioid Pain Relievers--United States, 19992008." *Mob Mortal Wily Rep 60*(43);1487-1492.

[119] Ibid.

[120] Grant M. "Danger Lurks with Used Transdermal Patches." *Pharmacy Times 78*(5): 34.

[121] National Poison Data System. 2016 Annual Report of the American Association of Poison Control Centers' National Poison Data System (NPDS): 34th Annual Report. Clin Toxicol (Phila). 2017.

[122] Agency for Healthcare Research and Policy. "Medication Errors and Adverse Drug Events." January 2019. Ahrq.gov.

[123] KFF.org. Henry J Kaiser Family Foundation.

[124] Ellen Gabler. "How Chaos at Chain Pharmacies is Putting Patients at Risk." *The New York Times*. January 31, 2020.

[125] Ibid.

[126] Jane Brody. "The Cost of Not Taking Your Medicine." *The New York Times*. April 17, 2017.

[127] Ibid.

Made in United States
North Haven, CT
04 November 2026

21766934R00183